PEOPLE-CENTRED PUBLIC HEALTH

Jane South, Judy White and Mark Gamsu

D0508728

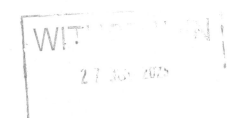
WIT...
2 7 ... ...

ACC: 308386
CLASS: WA 100 SOU

First published in Great Britain in 2013 by

The Policy Press
University of Bristol
Fourth Floor
Beacon House
Queen's Road
Bristol BS8 1QU, UK
t: +44 (0)117 331 4054
f: +44 (0)117 331 4093
tpp-info@bristol.ac.uk
www.policypress.co.uk

North American office:
The Policy Press
c/o The University of Chicago Press
1427 East 60th Street
Chicago, IL 60637, USA
t: +1 773 702 7700
f: +1 773-702-9756
e:sales@press.uchicago.edu
www.press.uchicago.edu

© The Policy Press 2013

British Library Cataloguing in Publication Data
A catalogue record for this book is available from the British Library.

Library of Congress Cataloging-in-Publication Data
A catalog record for this book has been requested.

ISBN 978 1 44730 530 9 (paperback)
ISBN 978 1 44730 531 6 (hardcover)

The right of Jane South, Judy White and Mark Gamsu to be identified as authors of this work has been
asserted by them in accordance with the 1988 Copyright, Designs and Patents Act.

All rights reserved: no part of this publication may be reproduced, stored in a retrieval system, or transmitted
in any form or by any means, electronic, mechanical, photocopying, recording, or otherwise without the
prior permission of The Policy Press.

The statements and opinions contained within this publication are solely those of the author and not
of the University of Bristol or The Policy Press. The University of Bristol and The Policy Press disclaim
responsibility for any injury to persons or property resulting from any material
published in this publication.

The Policy Press works to counter discrimination on grounds of gender, race, disability,
age and sexuality.

The Policy Press uses environmentally responsible print partners.

Cover design by Qube Design Associates, Bristol
Printed and bound in Great Britain by Hobbs, Southampton

FSC
www.fsc.org
MIX
Paper from
responsible sources
FSC® C020438

Contents

List of tables, figures and boxes

Tables

Figures

Boxes

Glossary

Citizenship: Citizenship is about people's active involvement in society, whether in a local, national or global context. Citizens have rights and responsibilities and they require the necessary knowledge and skills 'to understand, engage with and challenge the main pillars of our democratic society – politics, the economy and the law' (Citizen Foundation, 2012).

Commissioning: The process of ensuring that health and care services meet the needs of the population, including assessing population needs, prioritising health outcomes, contracting services and managing service providers (Turner and Powell, 2011).

Community: A group of people who share common characteristics, such as ethnicity, age, a shared interest (such as using the same service) or affinity (such as a shared faith), or other common bonds. A community can also be defined as a group of individuals living within the same geographical location (National Institute for Health and Clinical Excellence, 2008, p 38).

Community development: The process of 'building active and sustainable communities based on social justice, mutual respect, participation, equality, learning and co-operation' (National Institute for Health and Clinical Excellence, 2008, p 38). Community development involves challenges to existing power structures as people gain more control over their lives.

Community engagement: An umbrella term that is used to describe 'the process of getting communities involved in decisions that affect them. This includes the planning, development and management of services, as well as activities which aim to improve health or reduce health inequalities' (Popay, cited in National Institute for Health and Clinical Excellence, 2008, p 5).

Community health champion: Community health champions are individuals who are engaged, trained and supported to volunteer and use their understanding and position of influence to help their friends, families, neighbours or work colleagues lead healthier lives (Altogether Better, 2010).

Community health worker: Community health workers are recruited from local communities and carry out health care and/or prevention activities. They receive training and some support to deliver interventions, but do not have professional training (Lewin et al, 2005). Community health workers are sometimes called lay health workers or lay health advisors.

Community participation: 'The social process of taking part (voluntarily) in either formal or informal activities, programmes, and/or discussions to bring about a planned change or improvement in community life, services and/or resources' (Bracht and Tsouros, 1990, p 201).

Co-production: The shared design and delivery of services based on an equal and reciprocal relationship between professionals, people using services, their families, carers and neighbours (Boyle and Harris, 2009).

Empowerment: Concerns individuals and communities increasing control over their lives and is a central concept in health promotion. Individual empowerment is about individuals gaining a sense of control through increasing confidence, enhancing personal skills and developing coping mechanisms. Community empowerment is about allowing people to take control of the decisions that influence their lives and health (Wallerstein, 2006).

Health assets: The resources that 'people and communities have at their disposal, which protect against negative health outcomes and/or promote health status' (Morgan and Ziglio, 2007, p 18). This includes individual skills and knowledge, local organisations, and the environmental and economic resources in local communities.

Health inequalities: The differences in health and well-being between different groups that arise because of inequalities in social and economic conditions.

Health promotion: According to the World Health Organization (2009, p 1), health promotion is the process of enabling people to increase control over, and to improve, their health. Health is a positive concept, not merely absence of disease, therefore 'health promotion is not just the responsibility of the health sector, but goes beyond healthy lifestyles to wellbeing'.

Ideology: Ideology is a coherent body of interrelated ideas and values that underpins economic and political theory.

Lay health worker: Used in this book as a generic term to describe members of the public who take on roles within public health programmes but who do not receive professional or clinical training and are not employed as professionals.

Neoliberalism: A political movement based on the principles of free markets and individual freedom that favours relaxing economic regulation, increasing the role of the private sector, reducing the role of the state and promoting marketisation of public services.

Peer support: Peer support is the support provided and received by those who share similar attributes or types of experience. Peer support can be an informal process between people or can be provided through formal roles, where peer supporters seek to promote health and/or build people's resilience to different stressors (Dennis, 2003).

Primary Care Trusts: Local NHS organisations in England that have been (until 2013) responsible for commissioning health services, directing public health efforts within local districts and providing some community health services.

Public health: Public health aims to prevent disease, to improve health and well-being, and to reduce inequalities in health. It involves public policy combined with multi-sectoral action across the public, private and third sectors. Local communities and individuals have a key role to play in public health.

Public health system: A 'complex network of individuals and organisations that have the potential to play critical roles in creating the conditions for health' (US Institute of Medicine and Hunter et al, 2010, p 3). The public health system includes the resources and structures within government, public services (including health care), the third and private sectors, academia, the media, and communities, which can all act individually for health or together as a system.

Social action: The action taken to improve living and working conditions, promote justice, and combat inequality, building on the skills and experience of members of the public.

Social capital: 'Social capital is the degree of social cohesion in communities. It refers to the interactions between people that lead to social networks, trust, coordination and cooperation for mutual benefit' (National Institute for Health and Clinical Excellence, 2008, p 44). Social capital is described as 'bonding' where it refers to strong bonds within communities, 'bridging' where it refers to weaker links between communities and external organisations and groups, and 'linking' where there are connections across different levels of power or social status.

Social exclusion: Occurs when individuals, groups or whole communities are disadvantaged by exclusion from access to resources, services, democratic engagement and even basic human rights.

Systematic review: A research design that uses systematic and transparent research methods of literature searching, review and synthesis to assess the strength of the evidence on a specific topic.

Third sector: Used as an umbrella term to cover all not-for-profit organisations, including voluntary and community organisations, charities, social enterprises, cooperatives, and mutuals (HM Treasury and Cabinet Office, 2007). The term 'voluntary and community sector' is also used to describe the sector.

Volunteering: 'An activity that involves spending time, unpaid, doing something that aims to benefit the environment or individuals or groups other than (or in addition to) close relatives' (Volunteering England, 2012). Central to this definition is the fact that volunteering must be a choice freely made by each individual. It includes formal activity undertaken through public, private and third sector organisations as well as informal community participation.

Notes on the authors

Mark Gamsu is a Visiting Professor at Leeds Metropolitan University and has a strong interest in the relationship between citizenship, inequality and well-being. As well as freelance public health consultancy, he works part time for Health Action Partnership International, coordinating a European programme promoting Health in All Policies. As well as being on the board of a number of voluntary organisations in Sheffield, he is a Director of Citizens Advice. Mark has many years' experience in health and social care at community, district, regional and national levels, including leading on Joint Strategic Needs Assessments policy when working for the Department of Health. Mark runs a regular blog on citizenship and health (www.localdemocracyandhealth.com).

Jane South is Professor of Healthy Communities at the Institute for Health and Wellbeing, Leeds Metropolitan University, where she leads a research programme that links research, education and public engagement around the theme of community health and active citizenship, with a focus on lay health workers and volunteer roles in public health. Jane started her professional life as a nurse, moving into health promotion research 15 years ago, and later becoming Director of the Centre for Health Promotion Research at Leeds Metropolitan, where she has built a portfolio of community health research and publications, along with developing planning and evaluation frameworks for public health practice. Jane is currently working with local community organisations to establish a Community–Campus Partnerships for Health initiative.

Judy White is a Senior Lecturer in Health Promotion at Leeds Metropolitan University and Director of Health Together, a newly formed university enterprise for community engagement policy, practice and evidence. She is actively engaged in the Centre for Health Promotion Research, leading on a number of evaluations of health trainers and community health champions. Prior to taking up an academic post, Judy worked in the voluntary and community sector for 10 years and then in public health within the NHS for 22 years, where she had an interest in participatory approaches, establishing several health promotion programmes in Bradford. She continues to be the regional lead for health trainers and a key member of the national Health Trainer network.

Acknowledgements

People-centred public health is part of the Evidence for Public Health Practice series, which aims to provide an evidence-based resource of information on current policy and practice frameworks and to promote effective practice for key public health issues in the UK. The authors would like to thank The Policy Press and the series editors, Stephen Peckham and David Hunter, for their encouragement and guidance in developing this book.

The book draws extensively on findings from the People in Public Health study (2007–09), which was funded through the National Institute of Health Research (NIHR) Service Delivery and Organisation (SDO) Programme (project number 08/1716/206). This funding, originally part of a themed programme of public health research, created a genuine opportunity to undertake independent research into models in public health practice and ways of supporting lay engagement. The views and opinions expressed in this book are those of the authors and do not necessarily reflect those of the NHS, the NIHR or the Department of Health.

People in Public Health was a collaborative project, conducted in partnership with Bradford and Airedale teaching Primary Care Trust and the Regional Public Health Group, Government Office for Yorkshire & Humber. We would like to acknowledge the contribution of all members of the steering and advisory groups, research and administration teams, and other partners to that research. A number of individuals had major roles in carrying out data collection and analyses that informed the book and we would specifically like to thank:

- Martin Purcell and Rebecca Jones, for producing illuminating, high-quality case study reports for the Community Health Educators and Walking for Health projects, respectively.
- Karina Kinsella, for her excellent case study reports on the sexual health outreach and neighbourhood health projects, and for her role as the 'memory bank' of the project, which helped us with accuracy when we were writing up the book.
- Angela Meah, for all her work on the study, but particularly the literature review, which helped us understand different approaches and models.
- Peter Branney, for his creative ideas and critical analysis of public health practice.

This book contains many examples and resources from practice. We would like to acknowledge and thank the following for allowing us to use their material:

- Altogether Better, for use of Figure 2.1, 'The Altogether Better empowerment model'
- Jan Smithies and Georgina Webster, for use of their model presented in Figure 10.1: 'Essential elements of a community development strategy'
- Leeds Healthy Living Network, for details of their Community Health Educator course

- Sheffield NHS, for the case study of commissioning for community engagement.

In addition, we would like to thank Emily South, who took control of the book's reference material and spent many hours carefully checking, cross-referencing and correcting.

Finally, this book came about because we wanted to stimulate thinking on how the public could be more involved in public health. We have been privileged to listen to many people's experiences, both lay and professional, which continue to be a source of inspiration. What people do at the 'front line' of public health, often from within and alongside disadvantaged communities, is remarkable, and the value of that contribution undoubtedly deserves greater recognition.

Foreword

The Commission on the Social Determinants of Health 'Closing the gap in a generation' was commissioned by the World Health Organization and reported in 2008. The overarching recommendations included: improving daily living conditions for all people throughout life; tackling the inequitable distribution of power, money and resources; and measuring and understanding the problem and assessing the impact of action to achieve greater health equity in a generation.

Fair society, healthy lives (The Marmot Review, 2010a, 2010b) brought together the best available evidence and proposed six key policy objectives to address the social determinants of health and reduce the health gap in England. The report is clear. The underpinning objective is to create the conditions within which individuals and communities have greater control over their lives and greater political influence. Empowerment of individuals and communities was identified as an essential part of addressing the avoidable and, therefore, unjust inequalities that drive health inequalities, poor health and health behaviours.

Extending local democracy and giving people and local communities a greater say is driven by values of equity and social justice. This requires a shift in the culture of public health and public service away from deficit models to a more citizen-focused and asset-based approach that seeks to mobilise local capacity, contribution and creativity in defining and developing local solutions to local problems.

In the current global recession, there is a danger of a narrowing of focus, with prioritisation of the most vulnerable and attempts to do this with fewer resources. Such economic difficulties are not, however, a reason for inaction on health inequalities. Investment in early years, active labour market policies, social protection, housing and place, and the mitigation of climate change provide public protection and lay the foundations for a healthier future.

Radical reform is needed to transform the way in which services are designed and provided, taking upstream approaches that are people-centred in a whole-population perspective, which complements remedial work with early intervention and prevention focused on extending the resilience, capacity and capability of local people.

This publication sets out the main issues in developing and delivering such an approach. The focus is on creating a more collaborative framework within which co-production of health and well-being is secured on a more equitable basis between individuals, communities and public health services, facilitating community action on the social determinants of health.

Professor Sir Michael Marmot
Director
Institute of Health Equity
University College London

Dr Mike Grady
Principal Advisor
Institute of Health Equity
University College London

Series editors' preface

Health systems are changing rapidly in response to significant pressures on public finances and to neoliberal support for strengthening markets and competition, in addition to new threats to population health from lifestyle diseases, long-term conditions and the global effects of climate change. Public health as a set of skills to improve health, with its focus on the health of communities rather than individuals, is at the forefront of health policy and practice. In England, public health is going through a major transformation with local public health functions being returned to local government after nearly 40 years of being part of the NHS, and a new national public health service – Public Health England – being created. The coalition government's proposals for reorganisation, set out in the Health and Social Care Act 2012, introduce substantial uncertainty about roles and responsibilities in the new system and establish a different and challenging context for developing working relationships and partnerships. While the public health changes have been broadly welcomed by many, there remain reservations about how the new system will operate in a context of fiscal stringency. There are risks combined with anxiety and insecurity among many working in public health who are required to transfer from the NHS to local authorities. Whatever transpires, developing the new public health system places enormous challenges on those who will lead it and also those working within it.

This series of books on public health policy and practice aims to illuminate and inform thinking about many of the core issues to which the changes are directed, to add to the knowledge base for UK public health, and to address gaps in evidence and existing practice skills. The series has its roots in the publication of the Wanless Report (Wanless, 2004), the Cooksey Report (Cooksey, 2006) and a programme of research funded through the National Institute of Health Research (NIHR) Service Delivery and Organisation (SDO) Programme – now called the Health Services and Delivery Research programme. Cooksey identified the SDO Programme as filling an 'R&D market gap' and, therefore, as being of fundamental importance to the National Health Service (Cooksey, 2006). Following publication of the Cooksey Report, the Department of Health published Best research for best health (2006), and the government specifically highlighted the need for the SDO Programme to commission research on public health service delivery and organisation. The SDO Programme initially commissioned Professor David Hunter to undertake a review of the state of the public health system in England in terms of its structure, capacity and skills, and the likely impact of the current changes in policy in health and local government on the public health system and their implications for its future design and effectiveness (Hunter et al, 2010). The results of this review formed the background to the commissioning of further research that addressed four key areas: governance and incentives for public health at a local level; workforce; evaluating models of public health delivery; and approaches to public and community involvement in public health – reflecting concerns raised in the Wanless Report. While commissioned in 2008, the results of this programme of research have clear implications for the development of public health services in the future. The subject of this book – people-centred public health – is perhaps of particular relevance given the Coalition government's rhetoric surrounding the Big Society, including a growing emphasis on managing long-term conditions through self-management and the use of lay health workers, as well as a growing role for the third sector in place of traditional public services.

This book, therefore, is the first in a series of texts that explore contemporary issues relevant to the delivery and organisation of public health. Further books will examine public health partnerships, commissioning public health, and public health in general practice. These will present the findings of projects commissioned by SDO but updated to reflect the current changed context following the coalition government's policy and organisational changes. However, it is hoped that the series will be extended with the publication of further books drawing on the work of the UKCRC Public Health Research Centres of Excellence and also the new NIHR School for Public Health Research.

This book is a timely examination of an important area of public health that explores the role of volunteers and the community in public health. As Jane South and her colleagues demonstrate, lay public health workers are not a new idea or even a new phenomenon in health systems. There has, however, been increasing interest in their role at an international level as well as within the UK. Yet, in official circles and in discussions of the public health workforce in the UK, lay health workers have not figured to any significant degree. Nonetheless, the last 10 to 15 years have seen the growth of national programmes such as Walking for Health (the subject of Chapter Six in this book), the Expert Patients Programme, Community Health Champions, the Health Trainer Programme, and many initiatives outside the health field such as Sure Start with a network of children and parents' centres and Home-Start, with a network of nearly 16,000 trained parent volunteers who support parents who are struggling to cope. The richness and variety of such voluntary action is a key feature of this book.

The work reported in *People-centred public health* represents a significant shift in emphasis in public health research, and in particular, discussions about the public health workforce, including its remit and skills. Drawing on familiar concepts of community health workers, volunteerism and voluntary action, the authors provide a rich and detailed examination of the role of the lay public health worker. The book draws together the literature and evidence on lay public health roles and uses this as a context for the findings from their SDO-funded research project.

The book raises important questions about lay health workers in terms of their role and impact. Are they an extension of state control – a form of 'soft police' commandeered into national programmes to persuade, monitor and cajole the unhealthy? Or are they part of a genuine community movement that takes control of the local health agenda and their own health? These issues are critically examined by the authors, drawing on the international literature and are also explored within the context of the four case studies presented in the book:

—

Walking for Health, sexual health outreach, Community Health Educators and neighbourhood health.

The need for good-quality reliable evidence on how to organise and deliver effective public health interventions and programmes remains a high priority. National and local policy makers are actively addressing new public health problems and developing effective measures for tackling these, which raises key questions about funding, governance, the workforce, evidence of effectiveness and, increasingly, ethics. The strength of this book lies in its combination of evidence drawn from the international literature and the detailed case study research supported by the SDO. Clear lessons for practice are offered, which it is hoped those charged with developing and supporting public health in the UK will find useful.

Professor Stephen Peckham
Centre for Health Services Studies
University of Kent

Professor David Hunter
Centre for Public Health and Policy
Durham University

August 2012

ONE

Introduction

The public health system forms a framework encompassing all the different sectors that contribute to the public's health (Hunter et al, 2010). Despite the undisputed place of communities within that system, the contribution of civil society to meeting health goals receives minimal attention within public health policy and practice in England. Instead, public health effort has tended to focus on gathering evidence and working through organisations primarily in the health sector to deliver interventions supported by specialist practitioners. Communities can end up defined by their problems and therefore become the deserving 'target' of public health interventions, rather than being seen as part of the solution. Yet, at a more abstract level, community as a resource and a setting for public health continues to have importance, and support for increased community participation in health is reflected in national and international public health policy (Secretary of State for Health, 2010b; Department of Health, 2011b; World Health Organization, 2011). The mismatch between theory, policy and practice leaves scope for greater understanding of how the rhetorical value of 'community' can be translated into pragmatic strategies for social action on health. This book concerns one strategy for community engagement: the involvement of members of the public in delivering public health programmes and related community services.

Lay health worker and other peer-based interventions have a place in public health practice, and have been applied in many international contexts. The active involvement of lay people in service delivery draws in experiential knowledge, enhances social support processes and improves connections between services and individuals (Dennis, 2003; Rhodes et al, 2007). In England, increased citizen involvement in planning and running services (Secretary of State for Communities and Local Government, 2008) has been linked to the personalisation of health and social services and the patient and public involvement agenda (Department of Health, 2005b, 2008b). Indeed, community engagement has been described as 'an embedded feature of government policy, an act of faith that now extends across all the political parties' (Campbell et al, 2008, p 6). Coalition policy on the Big Society has given renewed emphasis to volunteering, social action, localism and citizen empowerment (Cabinet Office, 2011), but since this is occurring within a period of fiscal crisis, it poses a risk that communities will become the fallback when state services shrink. As Hunter et al (2010, p 157) comment in the first book of this series, the 'extremely difficult, if not hostile economic conditions ... when coupled with the environmental and sustainable development challenges ... put enormous pressure on a drive for social justice and narrowing the gap'. So, if improvements in health equity are to be realised, the contribution of members of the public to health is an issue of critical importance for the public health system.

The book sets out to provide a comprehensive overview of major themes for policy and practice in relation to engaging members of the public in delivering public health programmes, primarily as volunteers, but also as paid lay health workers. The book draws on the findings of the People in Public Health study (see the Appendix) to provide contemporary insights into key debates around why, how and with what support people can move from being health consumers to active citizens who are able to make a valued contribution to health. The focus is on how people take on a public health delivery role within the English public health system, although many of the themes for policy and practice will have resonance throughout the UK and in international contexts. Where comments about policy or practice apply across the UK, this is made clear in the text. While keeping a 'critical edge', the book has been designed to enable the reader to understand the challenges and opportunities for public services in developing new, more equal, relationships with communities.

Why is active citizenship a key issue for 21st-century public health?

The 20th century saw major improvements in the health of the UK population, attributed in part to the establishment of a comprehensive welfare state and to the improvement of living and working conditions. Sadly, improvements in health have been accompanied by a widening health gap between the health of those who are better off and those who are poor or live in poor areas (Department of Health, 2003). Health inequalities are present across all population groups and across areas and affect people across their life course. The recent Strategic Review of Health Inequalities in England post-2010, led by Sir Michael Marmot, highlighted the problem of a social gradient in health, with unequal societies having worse health outcomes (The Marmot Review, 2010a, 2010b). These inequalities are seen as unjust because they are largely avoidable.

In public health research, there has been a focus on describing and understanding the problem of health inequalities, what Hunter et al (2010, p 157) call 'the tendency endlessly to analyse the problems rather than act on them', and there is scope for more emphasis on solutions. The Marmot Review (2010a) represents a call to action. The public health system cannot rely on exhorting individuals to live healthier, eat better or exercise more. In the previous decade, two strategic reviews conducted by Sir Derek Wanless presented a cogent set of economic arguments for greater patient and public engagement in health, concluding that a 'fully engaged society' is a prerequisite for better health outcomes (Wanless, 2002, 2004). Governments and statutory organisations have always placed more emphasis on professionally led interventions to improve health and well-being than on solutions designed and delivered by communities themselves. This is particularly true with regard to communities who experience the greatest inequalities. At best, the welfare state has failed to mitigate the effects of inequalities; at worst, it perpetuates an unfair distribution of resources in society. The book examines one solution to the challenge of health inequalities: how the gap can be bridged between those at risk of poor health and access to the resources necessary to support good health.

The imperative for public health action, combined with the challenges for governance of an increasingly fragmented (and shrinking) public sector (Hudson and Lowe, 2009), appear to be driving interest in the role of citizens in health. At an international level, recent developments in health policy have reflected a renewed emphasis on the centrality of community participation to achieving better population health. In 2011, the Rio Declaration, which emerged from the World Conference on Social Determinants of Health held in Brazil, placed participation and community leadership as one of five areas of global action (World Health Organization, 2011). Signatories pledged to 'consider the contributions and capacities of civil society to take action in advocacy, social mobilization and implementation on social determinants of health' (World Health Organization, 2011, para 12.2 (v)). Harnessing the skills, knowledge and resources of lay people within public health programmes fits with this high-level statement. In 'Health 2020', the emergent European policy for health, increasing participation is one of six policy goals (World Health Organization Regional Office for Europe, 2012). Governance is a major theme of Health 2020, and a linked study, conducted as part of the policy development process and led by Ilona Kickbusch highlighted the need for new models of governance that accord a greater role to citizens, patients and consumers both in policy making and in individual health and care relationships (World Health Organization Regional Office for Europe, 2011). This book explores the need for local action to exist alongside structural solutions. It starts from the premise that there is potential for services to have a better fit with needs, but this is unlikely to happen without better relationships between communities and services. This involves challenges to those holding power and these themes will be explored in the book. It will demonstrate how people can make more of a difference to public health if they are involved as citizens rather than as passive recipients of public services.

The challenge of participation

Community participation, community engagement, patient and public involvement, citizen engagement, social action – these terms and their variants are all important concepts for public health policy and practice (see Glossary). Bracht and Tsouras (1990, p 201) define citizen participation as: 'The social process of taking part (voluntarily) in either formal or informal activities, programmes, and/ or discussions to bring about a planned change or improvement in community life, services and/or resources'.

The Declaration of Alma-Ata in 1978 stated that 'the people have the right and duty to participate individually and collectively in the planning and implementation of their health care' (World Health Organization, 1978). The World Health Organization has continued to endorse community participation as an essential element of health promotion and as a human right (World Health Organization, 2009). The World Health Organization Europe (World Health Organization, 2002) report on community participation approaches and techniques for local health and sustainable development summarises the different rationales for community participation as follows:

- To increase democracy as participation is a right and an essential element of citizenship;
- To combat social exclusion by giving people a voice, especially marginalised populations;
- To empower individuals and communities and enable them to gain more control over their lives;
- To mobilise community resources and energy;
- To develop holistic integrated approaches;
- To aid decision-making and design more effective services;
- To ensure community ownership and ultimately sustainability of programmes. (World Health Organization, 2002, pp 12–13)

Participation denotes citizens taking an active rather than passive role in their health and the health of their communities. New co-production models of governance advocated within Health 2020 show citizen involvement in both policy and individual spheres, so that the 'whole-of-society' approach is complemented by 'collaborative, communicative relationships' between individual patients and professionals (World Health Organization Regional Office for Europe, 2011, p 12). The purpose of engagement, the intensity of involvement and the range of participatory methods (participatory appraisal, citizens' juries, representative structures, lay advocacy, consultation techniques etc) will differ with each social context. In 2008, the National Institute for Health and Clinical Excellence (NICE) issued 'Guidance on Community Engagement', which acknowledged the diversity of methods, the difficulty in distinguishing terms and the potential for involvement with varying levels of power-sharing. The guidance chose the term 'community engagement' as an 'umbrella' term to describe: 'the process of getting communities involved in decisions that affect them. This includes the planning, development and management of services, as well as activities which aim to improve health or reduce health inequalities' (National Institute for Health and Clinical Excellence, 2008, p 5). It included recommendations to recruit community members as 'agents of change' 'to plan, design and deliver health promotion activities and help address the wider social determinants of health' (National Institute for Health and Clinical Excellence, 2008, p 28).

Recruiting lay health workers to become involved in the delivery of public health programmes, which is the subject of this book, is therefore one of a family of community engagement approaches. As suggested by Figure 1.1, mechanisms that serve to connect communities with public health systems and services operate at different levels, spanning from governance and planning through to delivery and public health intelligence, but often there are synergistic connections between involvement activities. As Figure 1.1 shows, citizen roles may also vary in terms of formality and independence, from natural helpers demonstrating neighbourliness through to formal lay representation on statutory bodies.

Any analysis of participation, whether at a theoretical, methodological or practical level, brings the concept of power to the fore. The extent to which participatory processes engender a shift in power from the state to society, from professional to lay, is the subject of much academic and political debate and these debates are alluded to at various points in the book. Empowerment has been described simply as a process by which 'people, organizations and communities gain mastery over their affairs' (Rappaport, 1987, p 122). Individual and community empowerment are seen as linked in a continuum of involvement that moves from individuals gaining more confidence and control over their health to collective action to address social injustice (Laverack, 2004; Wallerstein, 2006). While lack of power and low social status are associated with entrenched health inequalities (Wilkinson and Pickett, 2009), interventions that result in individuals and communities gaining greater control over their health are linked to better health outcomes and more equitable services (National Institute for Health and Clinical Excellence, 2008). Morgan (2001, p 221) highlights the 'definitional divide' between utilitarian models seeking to utilise community resources as a means to an end and empowerment models where participation is sought as an end in itself. In practice, the distinction between an instrumental use of participation and its constitutive value may not be that clear,

Figure 1.1: Citizen involvement in the public health system

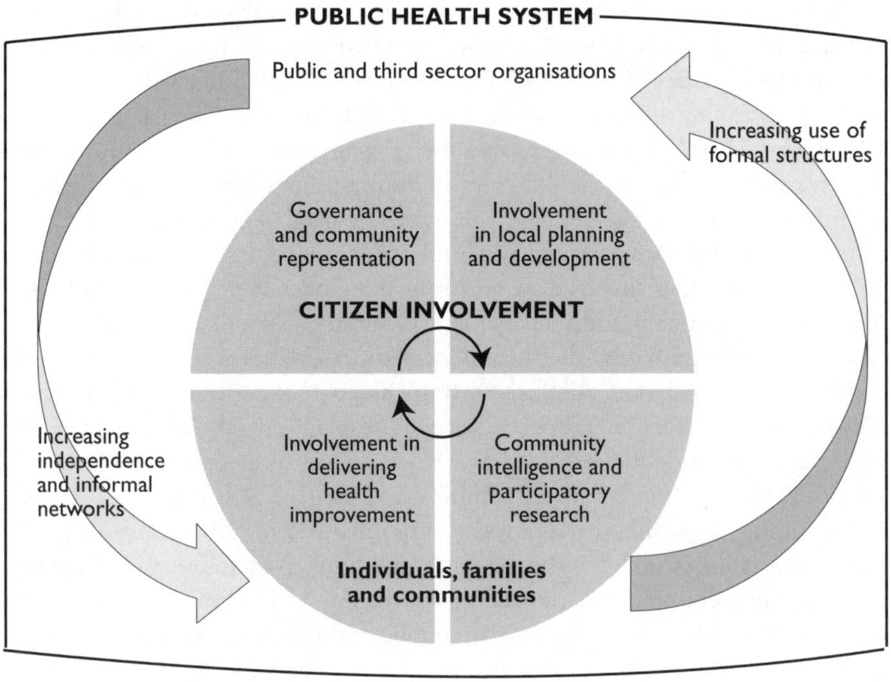

— **PUBLIC HEALTH SYSTEM** —

Public and third sector organisations

Increasing use of formal structures

Governance and community representation

Involvement in local planning and development

CITIZEN INVOLVEMENT

Increasing independence and informal networks

Involvement in delivering health improvement

Community intelligence and participatory research

Individuals, families and communities

as some of the case studies in the book highlight. Nonetheless, there needs to be a recognition that many participatory approaches are seeking reform and a more pluralistic style of delivery, rather than empowerment (Bridgen, 2004).

Citizen involvement can be problematic not only because of differing conceptual interpretations, but also because of the challenge to develop public health practice in a meaningful and effective manner. It is this gap between the aspiration of greater citizen involvement, reiterated in countless international and national policies, and the actuality of achieving even small shifts in practice that remains a persistent challenge. Just because action is justified does not mean it is easy to achieve. In England, there continue to be a plethora of initiatives that seek to establish co-produced relationships with citizens to improve health and well-being. Most of these do not achieve sufficient scale to challenge health systems, thereby ensuring long-term change. Even where there is good evidence of impact, there are barriers to transferring this knowledge into action. It is worth pausing to consider how many case studies of inspirational community health projects highlighting innovation have been showcased in policy documents and through national organisations' promotional material over the past 15 years. Yet, despite the overt support for involving communities, readers may wish to consider how few large-scale, well-resourced public health programmes that systematically involve communities exist in England.

The book discusses the practicalities of recruiting, training and supporting lay health workers and relates this to strategic approaches to tackling health inequalities. It also looks beyond the realm of the public health practitioner to discuss some of the broader issues around local impact and national influence. Many communities have been at the receiving end of community-based initiatives that operate from a 'deficit' approach (Foot and Hopkins, 2010); the idea being that if only people in communities are better educated, more aware, skilled and confident, then their problems would be sorted. This is often accompanied by professional lack of awareness of how services and public agencies operate to create and maintain unequal power differentials that result in barriers to engagement (South et al, 2009). Community-led approaches to improving health and well-being are frequently seen as interesting additions to the serious business of statutory commissioning and provision rather than a fundamental part of an engaged society. The book discusses the policy issues and barriers to engagement that operate at the micro, meso and macro levels. It seeks to provide some pointers to moving citizen involvement from the periphery to mainstream policy and practice.

Participatory ways of working will inevitably generate locally based, flexible solutions and, overall, this can present a messy picture where it is difficult to tease out the commonalities between approaches. People-centred ways of working do not usually set out to direct people along a predefined path or towards a particular set of behaviours, and this conflicts with the desire to produce neat political solutions to social problems. Rifkin et al (2000, p 37) explain that participation is not about linear and predictable change, but should be seen as an 'adaptive change mechanism'. The book provides readers with a critical guide to major

–

themes relating to citizen involvement as related to fundamental principles of public health practice, but does not endorse particular models.

Building a 'lay workforce' in public health

The idea that people can become leaders, motivators, educators and helpers around health issues in their communities is not new (see Chapter Three). There are people who do this naturally without the help of services and in many informal ways (Eng et al, 1997; The Commission on the Future of Volunteering, 2008). Community networks and informal systems of social support are key determinants of health (Wilkinson and Marmot, 2003; World Health Organization, 2011). At the same time, public services and third sector organisations can support this process through recruiting, training and supporting members of the public (lay people) to promote health. The role that people take on, the populations they work with and the activities they become engaged in vary considerably. Some examples of activities within public health practice are given in Table 1.1.

There is a confusing array of terminology to describe these lay roles. As explored further in Chapter Three, 'community health worker' (also known as 'lay health worker' or 'lay health advisor') is a generic term that has been applied across the world, although is rarely used in the UK. Community health workers (see Lewin et al, 2005; Rhodes et al, 2007; South et al, 2010b):

• are drawn from the target community;
• have not been trained as a health professional but receive some training to undertake the role; and

Table 1.1: Active citizens for health – examples of roles

Roles	Example of activities
Providing health information and simple advice.	– Talking to people in clubs and bars about the importance of sexual health screening and suggesting how they can go about getting tests.
Raising awareness of health issues.	– Distributing information to older neighbours on keeping warm in winter.
Improving skills.	– Running cook and eat sessions with parents and grandparents.
Providing peer support.	– Befriending new recruits to a green gym.
Promoting access to services or signposting.	– Using cultural and language skills to help women from minority ethnic groups get the right help in pregnancy and childbirth.
Facilitating community groups.	– Running a breastfeeding support group.
Supporting professional services.	– Welcoming and offering personal support to people attending a stop smoking clinic.
Organising and leading community-based activities.	– Leading health walks and exercise sessions.

Source: South et al (2010a, p 2).

• carry out a range of functions related to health promotion and health care in their communities.

There are also peer-based approaches, typically peer education, peer support and peer mentoring, which are based on lay health workers sharing characteristics, such as ethnicity or experience of long-term conditions, with the community of interest who they are working with. In addition to the involvement of lay people in formal public health interventions, volunteers carry out numerous roles in health and social care, both within the National Health Service (NHS) and other public services and working through voluntary sector organisations (Hawkins and Restall, 2006; Neuberger, 2008). The book describes some of the traditions of lay engagement, the core features of roles and the underpinning theories, as well as providing examples of different approaches in Chapters Three and Four.

In the UK over recent years, there has been a growing recognition of the lay contribution within a multidisciplinary public health workforce. As well as flagship programmes, such as the Expert Patient Programme (Department of Health, 2001a), Walking for Health (Natural England, 2011b) and the national Health Trainer programme (Department of Health, 2004, 2005a), approaches include befriending schemes, link workers, health advocates and community health champions as well as health promotion projects supported by volunteers (South et al, 2010b). The launch of the Public Health Skills and Career Framework helped bring about an acknowledgement of the place of lay workers and volunteers within the public health workforce. The framework describes the skills, knowledge and competencies of nine levels of public health practice from volunteer workers to public health leaders (Public Health Resource Unit and Skills for Health, 2008) (see Table 1.2). It extends the tripartite division set out in the Chief Medical Officer's report (Department of Health, 2001b) beyond the professional workforce to encompass lay workers and volunteers.

The context of a rapidly changing 'map' of the public health workforce led to the research study that has provided the framework for this book. The next section describes the People in Public Health study and its origin.

Table 1.2: Public Health Skills and Career Framework levels 1–3

	Level	Examples
Level 1	Has little previous knowledge, skills or experience in public health. May undertake specific public health activities under direction.	Volunteer workers (eg breastfeeding).
Level 2	Has gained basic-level public health knowledge through training and/or development. May undertake a range of defined public health activities under guidance.	Peer educator, lay health worker. Classroom assistant, refuse worker.
Level 3	May carry out a range of public health activities ... under supervision. May assist in training others and could have responsibility for resources used by others.	Community food worker, health trainer, dog warden, stop smoking advisor.

Source: Public Health Resource Unit and Skills for Health (2008, p 9).

–

The People in Public Health study

The idea of the book arose from the People in Public Health study (2007–09). This study was funded through the National Institute for Health Research (NIHR) and investigated approaches to develop and support lay people who take on public health roles. The NIHR Service Delivery and Organisation (SDO) programme (now the NIHR Health Services & Delivery Research Programme) had previously identified the need for a public health research stream, and public/community engagement was one of four work areas (Peckham et al, 2008). This book forms part of The Policy Press book series on public health edited by David Hunter and Stephen Peckham, which is based on a number of studies from this NIHR research programme.

The starting point for the People in Public Health study was the need for more evidence on how public services could develop and sustain community engagement to support better health outcomes. An earlier Home Office review had recommended more research to investigate both 'issues around people's willingness and capacity to become active citizens and issues around the willingness and capacity of public bodies to make best use of active citizens' (Rogers and Robinson, 2004, p 52). It was clear that there was scope for a review of approaches to involving lay people in public health roles. There were also identified gaps in knowledge regarding the experiences of lay health workers, the support role of health services and service-user perspectives.

The People in Public Health study sought to bring greater clarity around the different models in practice and to determine how public health services could support lay people involved in delivering public health programmes. The scope of the study was broad, but with a focus on interventions that aimed to reduce health inequalities or addressed the then public health priorities outlined in the White Paper *Choosing Health* (Department of Health, 2004). These were:

- reducing the number of people who smoke;
- reducing obesity and improving diet and nutrition;
- increasing exercise;
- encouraging sensible drinking;
- improving sexual health; and
- improving mental health.

There are a number of parallel fields of work that evidently contribute to public health that were not included in the study, such as peer support of parenting (eg Oakley et al, 2002) or peer-based approaches in the management of long-term conditions (eg Griffiths et al, 2007). The book has taken a broader perspective on lay health workers and made appropriate links to wider themes on the role of participation in health.

People in Public Health was based on a study design that drew on different sources of evidence, including published literature, practice-based evidence and lay perspectives (McQueen, 2001). Study methods included:

- a systematic scoping review of lay engagement in public health roles;
- three expert hearings where key informants with relevant expertise presented evidence on lay engagement;
- a Register of Interest collecting information about projects involving lay health workers; and
- five case studies of public health projects, which each reflected a different model of practice and community of interest. (Interviews were conducted with a total of 136 stakeholders including commissioners, practitioners, lay health workers and service users.)

The book draws on findings from across the People in Public Health study to illustrate points or provide practical examples. Four of the case studies have been written up as chapters in their own right. More details on the study methods and findings can be found in the Appendix, in the study report (South et al, 2010b) and on the study website,[1] which includes a searchable database of 224 publications on lay health workers (Bagnall, 2009) and a downloadable Research Briefing for practice (South et al, 2010a).

Definitions and meanings

The whole field of community participation is littered with contested terms and shifting meanings (Hawe, 1994; Cornwall, 2008). There is a wide array of terms used to describe lay roles (see Box 1.1) and the nomenclature of academic literature tends to differ from terms in common use in practice. The book uses the term 'lay health worker' as a generic term to describe members of the public who take on roles within public health programmes but who do not receive professional or clinical training and are not employed as professionals. Typically, individuals will undertake some training for the role and may receive some ongoing support or supervision. Some receive some payment in their roles and some work in a voluntary capacity; however, the issue of rewards is complex and will be discussed later in Chapter Ten. Labels can be artificial and many contributing to the public health agenda would not recognise their 'health' role. The term 'lay' can have religious overtones, and is rarely used in practice (South et al, 2010b), yet the term 'lay health worker' does provide some specificity and is to be preferred to more ambiguous terms like 'community engagement'.

'Community' is perhaps the most contested term of all. It is used: as a normative term to denote a set of valued social relations; as a categorisation of a population or group; as a description of place; as a setting for activity; and as a form of collective action (Butcher, 1993; Hawe, 1994). The book uses the term 'community' as an umbrella term for civil society but the authors acknowledge that communities are rarely homogeneous (Banks, 2003). Commonly, there is a distinction made between communities of place (geographic communities) and communities of identity, although both are interdependent (Campbell et al, 2008).

Much of the focus of the book is on volunteering, which has been defined as 'an activity that involves spending time, unpaid, doing something that aims to benefit the environment or individuals or groups other than (or in addition to) close relatives' (Volunteering England, 2012). Not all lay health worker roles are unpaid, which adds complexity (for further discussion, see Chapter Ten). There is also an important distinction to be made between individual citizens, whose participation may fluctuate from community leadership to non-participation (Taylor, 2003), and the voluntary and community sector. While voluntary organisations often provide a supportive infrastructure for citizen involvement, they are not synonymous with it, and volunteering occurs across both the statutory and third sectors. 'The third sector' is often used as an umbrella term to cover all not-for-profit organisations, including voluntary and community organisations, charities, social enterprises, cooperatives, and mutuals (HM Treasury and Cabinet Office, 2007). There is considerable diversity in the sector, from small user-led groups run by a handful of members to large, corporate-style charities (HM Treasury, 2002), with the balance of lay–professional interests and the proportion of volunteers (unpaid) to paid staff varying between organisations (Hogg, 1999). In addition, it should be remembered that many members of the public are engaged in public health activities (either as volunteers or paid lay health workers) through statutory public services, including the NHS (Hawkins and Restall, 2006).

Box 1.1: Examples of terms used to describe lay health worker roles

- Activators
- Community health educators
- Community health advocates
- Community health champions
- Community mobilisers
- Community nutrition assistants
- Lay health advisors
- Lay food and health workers
- Linkworkers
- Peer counsellors
- Peer coaches
- Peer educators
- Peer supporters
- Popular opinion leaders

- Outreach workers
- Volunteers

Source: South et al (2010b).

Values

The book has emerged from the authors' experiences of practice, research and policy development. We started the journey of evidence generation, exploration and critique from a shared value base; we believe in the importance of the lay contribution and that community participation both has an intrinsic value and is a mechanism to achieve better health. We also believe in equity and social justice and endeavour to explore how these might be achieved in a modern welfare state that faces seemingly intractable problems not just in relation to resources, but in terms of serious health issues that can blight people's lives. The book argues that citizen involvement has to be part of a strategic response that includes healthy public policy and reorientation of health care services, following the principles of the Ottawa Charter for health promotion (World Health Organization, 1986).

The authors' experiences suggest that good, high-quality services will value community engagement and that organisations can best serve people by being in touch with their needs and aspirations. While acceding that the lay contribution is a vital element of public health, the book also provides some critical analysis of policy, evidence and practice. Involving people in service delivery is about power shifts and system change and it is not helpful to gloss over issues of effectiveness, equity and managerial challenges. Not all solutions will be successful; neither can it be assumed that radical solutions are always preferable to small reforms. This means that the book explores a variety of ways of involving people and does not shy away from discussing some of the dilemmas and challenges that occur in practice. The intention is to broaden understandings and stimulate debate rather than provide an expert view. In the context of the major changes facing society, the book critiques some of the traditional ways of thinking in public health and presents fresh ideas for developing new roles for citizens.

Structure of the book

Chapter Two looks at the policy context in which citizen involvement is promoted, and sometimes constrained. The chapter provides an overview of current policy on volunteering and social action, looking at the contribution of volunteering to society and the significance of active citizenship within broader calls for democratic renewal. The concept of the Big Society, which has been adopted as a central idea within Coalition policy, is discussed in the context of the retrenchment of public services. Major themes pertaining to community engagement that thread through health and public health policy in England are introduced and policy conflicts are highlighted.

Chapter Three gives an overview of lay health workers, where the concept originated and the traditions that have emerged internationally in both the global South and North America, providing case studies and examples. The chapter aims to provide a context for understanding the lay health worker models that have been developed in the UK and descriptions are provided of major initiatives such as the Expert Patient Programme and health trainers. Consideration is given to independent community-initiated action on health and how this relates to more professionally directed programmes.

Chapter Four discusses the main justifications for citizen involvement in public health. It presents six reasons for involving members of the public in delivering health improvement drawn from the People in Public Health study, and discusses these in relation to theory, research and practice. The evidence base for lay health workers is briefly reviewed, along with a discussion of economic and moral arguments. It concludes that a better understanding of the individual, social and organisational benefits that can result from citizen involvement is needed.

Chapter Five reports on lay perspectives, drawn mainly from interviews with lay health workers and service users in the People in Public Health study, but also drawing on evidence from community health champion programmes. The chapter looks at motivations for being a volunteer, barriers to joining and progressing, gaining life skills, and pathways to personal development, employment and education. Perspectives on lay skills and qualities are explored and the chapter argues that lay health workers bring valuable life experience, local knowledge and an empathy with their community that allow them to carry out public health roles.

Chapters Six to Nine present detailed case studies of public health projects involving lay people that were conducted as part of the People in Public Health study. Based on interviews with commissioners, managers, project staff, lay health workers and, in some cases, service users, the case studies provide insights into what public health programmes involving lay health workers look like in real-life contexts and illuminate some of the dilemmas and strengths of working in this way. **Chapter Six** deals with volunteer engagement in a local Walking for Health scheme. It discusses the role and responsibilities of volunteer walk leaders and the need for programme support and coordination. **Chapter Seven** presents findings from a small sexual health outreach project using volunteers to support the delivery of a community-based screening service aimed at men who have sex with men. The chapter highlights some interesting issues about boundaries and how risk was managed. **Chapter Eight** concerns a community health educators programme, where the lay health workers performed a bridging role working with disadvantaged communities. This case study provides an interesting example of where lay workers received payment rather than working as volunteers. A case study of a neighbourhood health project based in a disadvantaged housing estate is presented in **Chapter Nine**. High levels of participation were evidenced and the chapter discusses sustainability and the advantages and pitfalls of moving to greater citizen control.

Chapter Ten looks at how lay health worker programmes can be commissioned, developed and managed. It identifies common challenges as well as discussing strategies to enhance the experience of those volunteering or working as lay health workers. The chapter explores the need for effective leadership and management and argues for the adoption of new commissioning models that recognise the benefits of citizen involvement in service delivery.

Chapter Eleven attempts to provide counter-arguments to some of the common 'myths' about citizen involvement. It is intended to raise important questions about the place of lay engagement in society and provoke debate. The chapter looks at some of the ideological perspectives on involvement and volunteering from both the Left and Right of the political spectrum. Perceived threats to jobs and professionalism are explored and alternative perspectives are offered. The chapter also discusses the evidence base for lay health workers and the politics of evaluation.

Chapter Twelve summarises the major themes of the book. It reiterates the need to deliver public health differently in order to address health inequalities and to improve health in a sustainable way. Engaging with lay people and communities has to be central to the redesign of health services and form part of a fresh approach to public health. The book ends with a manifesto for a 'citizen-centred public health system'.

Note

[1] See www.leedsmet.ac.uk/health/piph/

TWO

The policy context

In response to the fiscal and political challenges facing society, governments have been prompted to re-evaluate the relationship between citizens and the state and, at least within policy documents, to recognise the contribution that the public can make to health and social care. This chapter examines the current policy context, and traces some of the major policy themes concerning citizen involvement in service delivery. It looks at how the rhetoric of some policies is in sharp contrast not just with other policy pronouncements, but also with the actions taken by government.

The chapter starts by briefly sketching the scale of contribution of current volunteering. In doing this, it notes that volunteer activity is very often happening independent of state activity, although, at the same time, it is true that the scale and coverage of voluntarism can be affected by government policy. There is a discussion on why successive governments have become interested in volunteering and community engagement, with a particular focus on the current Coalition government's Big Society initiative (Cabinet Office, 2010). The most recent Department of Health policy on volunteering (Department of Health, 2011b) and government support for The Marmot Review (2010a) on health inequalities are contrasted with mainstream National Health Service (NHS) policy. While the focus of this chapter is on volunteering, it is important to note that some lay roles are paid, in particular, health trainers, a new public health workforce introduced by the Labour government (see Chapter Three).

The New Economics Foundation (NEF) and National Endowment for Science, Technology and the Arts (NESTA) have put forward new ways of thinking about the state, its relationship with citizens and how health and social care could be provided in a more equitable and empowering way (Ryan-Collins et al, 2007). The chapter concludes that a different model of public health is needed, an argument that is developed further in the conclusion (Chapter Twelve).

Volunteering in England

The contribution of volunteers and members of the public (lay people) to society as a whole is substantial. Over the last 20 years, there has been a growing interest in understanding the scale of volunteering, what motivates people to do it, its benefits and how volunteer activity relates to the roles of the market and the state. Much of this research has been commissioned at the heart of the government, primarily by the Cabinet Office through the Office for Civil Society, and delivered by organisations such as the Institute for Volunteering Research and Volunteering England.

The research on volunteering shows that the social and economic contribution volunteers make is considerable. In October 2011, the Department of Health strategic vision for volunteering (Department of Health, 2011b, p 15) noted that:

- formal volunteering contributes approximately £21.5 billion to the UK economy each year (based on estimates from the National Council for Voluntary Organisations);
- when informal activity is factored in, volunteers may contribute around £48.1 billion to the economy annually (based on estimates from Volunteering England); and
- around 3.4 million people volunteer in health (based on estimates from Skills for Health).

For comparison, the total funding invested by the Treasury in the NHS is approximately £106 billion (2011/12). Similarly, the Cabinet Office Commission on the Future of Volunteering (Institute for Volunteering Research and Volunteering England, 2007, p 6) gave an example of a pilot survey of 59 hospices which found that for each £1 spent on supporting volunteers, hospices received a return of more than £11. The conclusion was: 'if hospices had to pay for staff to do the work contributed by volunteers, their running costs would increase by nearly a quarter'.

While the volunteer contribution to health and social care is substantial, it is important to bear in mind that volunteers make a wider and arguably more significant contribution to health and well-being through activity outside the sector that has a direct impact on the social determinants of health. A national survey carried out for the Cabinet Office by the National Centre for Social Research and the Institute for Volunteering Research (Low et al, 2008, p 25) shows that volunteers are involved across a wide range of organisations, as shown in Table 2.1. Volunteering is not just good for society as a whole, but also for the individuals concerned (Casiday et al, 2008), and this topic is explored further in Chapter Five.

The Institute for Volunteering Research and Volunteering England (2007, p 4) suggest a useful taxonomy for understanding the range of volunteering:

- Mutual aid or self-help – people with shared problems, challenges or conditions working together to address them.
- Philanthropy or service to others – most commonly, volunteering through a voluntary or community organisation to provide some form of service to one or more third parties or beneficiaries.
- Participation – the involvement of individuals in the political, governance or decision-making process at any level.
- Advocacy and campaigning – collective action in formal or informal groups, or as individuals, to secure or prevent change.

—

Table 2.1: Types of organisations helped by volunteers

Sector	All respondents (%)	Current volunteers (%)
Education – schools, colleges, universities	18	31
Religion	14	24
Sports, exercise	13	22
Health, disability	13	22
Children, young people	11	18
Local community, neighbourhood, citizens' groups	10	17
Hobbies, recreation, social clubs	8	13
Overseas aid, disaster relief	6	11
Animal welfare	6	10
Elderly people	5	8
Arts and museums	5	8
Conservation, the environment and heritage	4	8
Social welfare	4	7
Politics	2	4
Safety, first aid	2	4
Justice, human rights	2	4
Trade unions	2	3
Other	2	3

Source: Low et al (2008, p 25).

This book focuses on the first two types of volunteering and how members of the public contribute to improving public health, while also recognising that initial engagement in helping others can lead to participation more generally or to lobbying for changes that address the determinants of ill health and inequality.

Government and volunteering

Successive governments since the 1970s have acknowledged that volunteering is an important part of the way people engage with society. In her introduction to the Commission on the Future of Volunteering report on volunteering and social policy (Institute for Volunteering Research and Volunteering England, 2007, p 3), Baroness Julia Neuberger notes that:

> In the last twenty years government has recognised the critical contribution that volunteering makes to building a strong and cohesive society. It has promoted volunteering as 'the essential act of citizenship', a means for combating social exclusion, and an important contributor to the delivery of high quality public services.

One of the key reasons for the growing governmental interest in volunteering in this country has been concerns about the 'democratic deficit', that is, the disengagement of people from the democratic process and civic institutions in general. From a US perspective, Alinksy and McKnight (cited in Community Sector Coalition, 2010, p 2) argue that the link between social action and democracy is critical:

> The heart of democracy is the free space where people form their own associations to provide care, advocacy and community. Without this vital centre, democracies become hollow and institutions become oppressive and unresponsive. And people lose their citizenship by becoming nothing more than clients and consumers.

There has been growing unease about the relationship between the state and the individual, and concern that an over-reliance on state services can disempower individuals and remove responsibility. This has been coupled with the recognition that existing solutions to address 'wicked issues', such as health inequalities, have not worked (The Marmot Review, 2010a). Add to this a body of evidence supporting a shift in focus to upstream prevention activity and a 'fully engaged' population if fiscal challenges in the health sector are to have any chance of being met (Wanless, 2002, 2004) and it is easy to see why there has been an interest in developing a more sophisticated narrative about the relationship between the active citizen and the state (Blunkett, 2003; Secretary of State for Communities and Local Government, 2008).

The policy problem has both a collective dimension and an individual dimension, focusing on the need for reform of the client–professional relationship (Neuberger, 1998; Sang, 2004). The last decade witnessed a shift in policy with considerably more prominence being given to the Patient and Public Involvement agenda in the health sector (NHS Executive, 1999; Department of Health, 2001b, 2001d, 2005b) and a broader notion of community involvement threading through policies in regeneration, social care and local government (Social Exclusion Unit, 2001; Department for Education and Skills, 2002; Communities and Local Government, 2007; Campbell et al, 2008). The result was a complex web of interlinked policies that both initiated reforms in the governance and organisation of the public sector and attempted to refine the role of the citizen in creating better communities and neighbourhoods. Examples included:

- the 'Neighbourhood Renewal Strategy', which identified a key role for communities in improving disadvantaged neighbourhoods (Social Exclusion Unit, 2001);
- *Shifting the balance of power*, which set out the primary functions of primary care groups, advocating for a shift in power towards front-line staff and local communities (Department of Health, 2001d, 2002);
- *Tackling health inequalities: a programme for action*, which identified 'Engaging Communities and Individuals' as one of four interlinking themes (Department of Health, 2003);

- the Local Government and Public Involvement in Health Act 2007, which created Local Involvement Networks to support the user voice in health services and mandated local authorities to work with Primary Care Trusts to undertake joint strategic needs assessments of heath needs; and
- the White Paper *Our health, our care, our say*, which argued for greater personalisation of care and increased patient influence (Secretary of State for Health, 2006).

The need to develop a new paradigm in response to concerns about the democratic deficit and the relationship between public services and citizens started to appear more clearly in policy documents that emerged towards the end of the Labour government led by Gordon Brown (2008–10). Hazel Blears, who was then Secretary of State for Communities and Local Government, advocated the need to rebalance power from the state towards communities and individuals in a key policy document, *Communities in control: real people, real power* (Secretary of State for Communities and Local Government, 2008, p 1):

> We want to shift power, influence and responsibility away from existing centres of power into the hands of communities and individual citizens. This is because we believe that they can take difficult decisions and solve complex problems for themselves. The state's role should be to set national priorities and minimum standards, while providing support and a fair distribution of resources.
>
> A vibrant participatory democracy should strengthen our representative democracy. The third sector – through charities, voluntary organisations and social enterprises – has much to offer from its traditions of purposeful altruism and selfless volunteering. Equally, we believe that political activity is a worthwhile and essential part of British life, and we want to restore people's faith in politics.

The Labour government had insufficient time to translate their aspirations into policy reforms before they lost power in 2010, but similar ideas and concerns underpin the development of the concept of the Big Society, which has been central to the policy of the Coalition government elected in 2010. Prime Minister David Cameron has attempted to place what is essentially his project at the heart of government policymaking with the aim of redefining the relationship between the citizen and the state (Box 2.1), describing it as a 'different way of going about trying to change our country for the better' (Cameron, 2011).

Box 2.1: The Big Society

The Cabinet Office was given responsibility for taking forward the work of the Big Society, which is described as follows: 'The Big Society is about helping people to come together to improve their own lives. It's about putting more power in people's hands – a massive transfer of power from Whitehall to local communities.'

There are three key elements of the Big Society agenda:

- community empowerment: giving local councils and neighbourhoods more power to take decisions and shape their area;
- opening up public services: public service reforms to allow third sector organisations and private companies to tender to deliver welfare services; and
- social action: encouraging and enabling people to play a more active part in society.

There are deliberately few national policy directives associated with the Big Society, but some national initiatives, for example, the National Citizen Service for 16 year olds and Community Organisers, have been established with the aim of encouraging 'people to get involved in their communities'.

Source: Cabinet Office (2011).

The Big Society has been described as a slippery concept and a 'Big Con' because it simplifies the complex relationships between the state and citizens to a single direction of travel towards a smaller state (Hunter, 2011). Despite Cameron's enthusiastic endorsement, the idea has struggled to gain momentum for a number of reasons. First, it has been resisted by many local authorities and citizen-led organisations on the basis that the Big Society community empowerment agenda masks cuts to central government funding, which inevitably leaves local organisations to pick up the pieces. Second, 'opening up public services' was perceived by many as a synonym for privatising public sector provision. Third, as is evidenced by the activity described in this book, social action has been flourishing without overt government support for a very long time, leading to considerable scepticism from within the voluntary and community sector about why the government was suddenly so interested. This has led to hesitancy by many to align themselves with the Big Society agenda. Finally, the concept of the Big Society has proved very difficult to pin down, as illustrated by Big Society Tsar Lord Nat Wei's description of it as:

> a coral reef represented by the many current and future providers of those [public] services that add variety and innovation and humanity to their delivery … it is the very fish that feed in these waters, the local citizen groups that can extend, vivify and shape this landscape in ambitious as well as humble ways. (Wei, 2010)

The concerns just outlined have been clearly articulated by a range of voluntary sector organisations and leaders. For example, in their publication *Unseen, unequal, untapped, unleashed*, the Community Sector Coalition (2010, p 4) argued that there are 'hundreds of thousands of community groups and millions of people who are involved in them' who are 'collectively taking action to address local issues in their communities'. Furthermore:

> At a time of massive cuts 'community resilience' is what will determine how well local people will survive. When there is no public sector money, when business retreats, all that is left is the collective action of ordinary people. The Coalition believes the scale of community action is not really recognised and understood. Community groups are often overlooked and ignored by government third sector policy. (Community Sector Coalition, 2010, p 3)

Their scepticism sadly became reality when the Community Sector Coalition lost its government funding at the end of March 2011 and made its three employees redundant. Many other voluntary and community groups have also had their funding reduced or discontinued, leading the National Council for Voluntary Organisations (NCVO Funding Commission, 2010) to say that they feared that, of the two future funding scenarios they paint, the one that sees third sector funding drastically reduced looks set to be the one that becomes reality (see Box 2.2).

Box 2.2: Two future funding scenarios

Under one scenario, the present pattern of public services is cut to the bone, serving fewer and fewer people. Commercial organisations take over the running of many of the services that are left, working to narrow eligibility criteria under large scale, performance-based contracts. The public sector protects its own. CSOs [civil society organisations] become hopelessly overstretched and unsustainable through reductions in their funding and an unrealistic assumption that voluntary effort and income can fill the gap left by the state's withdrawal. Disadvantaged communities suffer most and inequalities increase, as the cuts in public services and welfare benefits begin to bite.

Under another scenario, instead of steady decline, it is possible to envisage a radical shift through which the present pattern of public services and models for delivery are altered through co-production with service users. A new social contract is developed, involving innovative partnerships between the public, commercial and civil society sectors and new financing arrangements, including increased voluntary income. CSOs have stepped up to the mark to realise their full potential. Government investment and commercial sponsorship has helped CSOs do this. Local people and service users have played a central role in shaping the future.

Source: NCVO Funding Commission (2010, p 5).

The governmental response to the economic crisis has been to make large-scale public sector cuts (Cuts Watch, 2012), although the total welfare bill continues to rise with the growth in unemployment and rise in inflation (*The Telegraph*, 2011). The Coalition government has also embarked on the largest restructuring of the NHS in its history, a restructuring that Pollock and Price (2011) see as representing the end of the NHS as a universal service. The government has sought to distance itself from responsibility for cuts in front-line services by claiming that reductions in spending can be achieved by efficiencies, and through its localism agenda, laying responsibility on local government to make decisions about what to cut. The policy rhetoric on supporting local community-based activity can be seen to be at odds with the negative impact of the public sector cuts on public and third sector local organisations. Concerns have not been restricted to the voluntary sector or the opposition. In early 2011, the Public Administration Select Committee (2011), chaired by the Conservative MP Bernard Jenkin, initiated an investigation into the Big Society initiative, questioning the role for national and local government. So, two years into a Coalition government, the Big Society concept is greatly undermined by a neoliberal agenda concerned with cutting public services and opening the remainder up to the private sector. Its enduring rhetorical power is perhaps because it directs attention to some of the fundamental questions about the state–society relationship in a period of fiscal crisis. The right-wing think tank ResPublica (Wilson et al, 2011, p 3) argues that:

> The coming together of the big society agenda and huge public sector cuts has spawned a rare thing: a real public discussion about how we live, govern and solve problems. In the midst of this discourse there is one area of clear consensus; the call for big society demands more people getting involved in community life. However, it will not be easy to get people involved on the scale needed and this needs to be openly acknowledged.

ResPublica goes on to state that the key test will be what the government does to promote and strengthen volunteering, both through specific policies and initiatives, and additionally through cultural changes to mainstream policy and programmes which create a new environment that fosters voluntary action. The next section examines health policy on volunteering and how this fits (or not) with mainstream Department of Health and NHS policy.

Volunteering and the Department of Health

The Department of Health has long recognised the contribution that volunteering can make to the delivery of health and social care services, the empowerment of patients, and the improvement of public health (Department of Health, 2008b). Nonetheless, for a number of reasons, the approach taken has often appeared to be incoherent, small-scale and short-term. Foremost among the delivery challenges faced by the Department of Health is the continuing rise in the costs of health and social care, in large part caused by the demographics of an ageing population.

Linked to this is the challenge of how to support older people and disabled people to live longer and more independently in their own homes. For public health, the challenge remains how to narrow the gap between the health of the worst off and the better off, as measured by life expectancy and disability-free life years, and to halt the rise of non-communicable lifestyle-induced disease such as obesity and diabetes (Secretary of State for Health, 2010b).

The relationship between policymakers at the Department of Health, their delivery arms in the NHS and local authorities, who deliver adult social care, is complex. The NHS is a huge organisation, and has traditionally been a very obedient delivery arm of Department of Health policy. This close relationship, the scale of the NHS and its dominant clinical paradigm has inevitably shaped Department of Health priorities and how it seeks to deliver them towards a medical, rather than a social, model of health.

The Department of Health has a long-standing interest in volunteering and there are numerous practical examples of programmes and initiatives it has sponsored and commissioned; a number of which are detailed elsewhere in this book. The current Department of Health policy on volunteering is captured in its 2011 strategy document *Social action for well-being: building co-operative communities, Department of Health strategic vision for volunteering* (Department of Health, 2011b). This document is similar to the 'Strategic Vision for Volunteering' published a year and a half earlier under the previous Labour government (Department of Health, 2008b), but now reflecting the Coalition government's focus and language. It sets out the Department of Health's vision for volunteering in health and social care:

> Our vision is a society in which social action and reciprocity are the norm and where volunteering is encouraged, promoted and supported because it has the power to enhance quality, reduce inequality or improve outcomes in health, public health and social care. (Department of Health, 2011b, p 6)

This document details why the Department of Health considers volunteering and wider social action to be essential to health and social care, describing how it 'contributes to prevention, the creation of people-centred and relationship-based services and improved patient and service user experience' (Department of Health, 2011b, p 12). The vision recognises the multidimensional impact of volunteering for individuals (learning new skills, meeting other people, contributing new ideas, keeping people active, reducing social isolation) and the added value for organisations by improving outcomes and raising funds. In addition, the document identifies the contribution that volunteering can make to preventing ill health, reducing health inequalities and promoting public health, in particular, through the role that volunteer champions can play in helping people change their behaviour. The Department of Health is clear that the government's role in promoting social action is a facilitative one; nonetheless, it should 'remove bureaucratic barriers and promote the cultural change necessary for social action and voluntary activity to flourish' (Department of Health, 2011b, p 16). The document (Department of Health, 2011b, p16) sets out the intention to work with partners to:

- raise awareness of the potential for volunteering;
- improve the evidence base for investment; and
- increase access to best practice.

Given the strong relationship between health, well-being and volunteering (Casiday et al, 2008; Teasdale, 2008), it is unsurprising that the Department of Health has developed a vision for volunteering, but the real test of its value rests in how far it has impacted on mainstream policy within the NHS, adult social care and public health. It is noteworthy that in recent key health policy documents, there is virtually no mention of volunteering:

- In July 2010, the government published *Equity and excellence: liberating the NHS* (Secretary of State for Health, 2010a), which set out it future plans. There are no references to volunteering in this document.
- In November 2010, *Healthy lives, healthy people: our strategy for public health in England* (Secretary of State for Health, 2010b) was published. There are three references to volunteers in this document: one is concerned with a Department of Work and Pensions scheme aimed at the newly retired; one is in a case study; and one is about a programme led by the Department for Culture, Media and Sport for sports volunteers linked to the Olympics.
- In November 2010, the government published *A vision for adult social care: capable communities and active citizens* (Department of Health, 2010c). There are two references to volunteers in this document, one of which is concerned with giving front-line professionals more autonomy to develop working relationships with carers and volunteers.

While the primary focus of these policy documents is with the agenda to drive through major structural reform of the health system, it is nonetheless striking that references to volunteering are so sparse. It appears as though the debate about the Big Society led by the Prime Minister and driven through the Cabinet Office has barely touched mainstream health policy.

Public health policy and citizen involvement

Since 1974, and up until the recent Coalition health reforms, the public health function, with its three domains of health protection, health improvement and health services (Faculty of Public Health, 2012), has been based in the NHS, which has given the Department of Health significant managerial influence and an ability to ensure consistent practice. Department of Health public health policy has over the years placed a greater emphasis on actions that could either be addressed by NHS services and the professionals employed within them, through better targeted, higher-quality, more equitably available services, or through addressing the population as potential patients, providing them with information to enable them to make informed decisions about their health and well-being. Despite acknowledgement of the need for a multidisciplinary public health workforce (Department of Health, 2001c) and the opening up of consultant training to non-medics (PhORCAST, no date), public health leadership has remained dominated by clinically trained public health specialists; additionally, there has been a demise of health promotion specialists within public health (Scott-Samuel and Springett, 2007). The result has been that public health policy at both national and local levels has maintained a strong focus on NHS-led public health interventions and a tendency to follow a biomedical model, with less emphasis given to social determinants and citizen involvement.

From 1997 onwards, community engagement did become a key concept in much of the public health policy of successive Labour governments (Campbell et al, 2008), key examples including: *Saving lives: our healthier nation* (Secretary of State for Health, 1999); Health Action Zones (Department of Health, 1999; Sullivan et al, 2006); the *Choosing health* White Paper, which introduced health trainers (Department of Health, 2004); and *Tackling health inequalities: a programme for action* (Department of Health, 2003). While community engagement was a consistent and cross-cutting policy theme, the public health response to addressing health challenges like obesity and diabetes comprised three main elements:

- clinical interventions – such as improving access to screening and statins, access to specialist smoking cessation services, and encouraging health professionals to influence behaviours through brief interventions;
- health-promoting messages – through national programmes such as Change4Life; and
- patient empowerment – such as the establishment of the national Health Trainer Programme (Department of Health, 2005a) and the Expert Patient Programme (Department of Health, 2001a).

Superficially, this appears to be a balanced approach; however, historically, public health policy and funding have been weighted very heavily to the first two elements and, with a few notable exceptions, programmes based on citizen involvement have tended to be small-scale and marginal. As this book makes clear, less attention has been given to systematically involving the public in developing solutions to take greater control of their own health, particularly with regard to capitalising on the contribution that local government could make in facilitating this.

The Coalition health reforms, proposed in the 2010 White Paper *Equity and excellence: liberating the NHS* (Secretary of State for Health, 2010a) and enacted through the Health and Social Care Act 2012, introduce significant organisational changes for public health, and arguably these changes offer opportunities for more intensive and sustained community engagement. Local authorities will now

—

take the lead for public health and be responsible for coordinating local efforts to protect the public's health and well-being. Unusually, this is an aspect of the reforms that has been positively received in many quarters (Department of Health, 2011a), despite reservations about fragmentation, loss of independence and control of budgets (McKee et al, 2011). The reforms mean that local political leaders and elected members will have a much clearer responsibility for the health and well-being of their communities. Directors of Public Health, together with most of the public health workforce, will move from Primary Care Trusts to be based in local authorities. In order to encourage joined-up working at a local level, in particular, between the NHS and local government, there is a new duty on local authorities to establish Health and Wellbeing Boards (HWBs), which must include elected members, Clinical Commissioning Group representatives, Healthwatch and relevant local authority directors. At a national level, a new executive agency, Public Health England, will be created with wide-ranging responsibilities, including: health information and intelligence; population behaviour change through social marketing; building an evidence base; and supporting the development of the public health workforce.

The transfer of public health to local government undoubtedly presents opportunities for public health to spearhead the development of local policy and programmes based on stronger relationships with local communities. Despite ongoing concerns about the democratic deficit characterised by the comparatively low turnout at local elections, local councillors can still lay claim to being the commissioners who are closest to communities. Many live alongside the people they represent, are accountable to them through elections and public meetings, and talk to them in their surgeries. The closeness and longevity of this relationship with elected members creates a different culture to that of the NHS. At its best, local government from the top down is entwined with the community it serves and, as the previous government's *Communities in control* White Paper (Secretary of State for Communities and Local Government, 2008) highlighted, local authorities are used to engaging with people in various ways: as council taxpayers; as consumers of services; as volunteers; as active citizens with ambitions for changing local conditions; as local leaders; and as community representatives. The local authority culture and processes within local government therefore provide a real opportunity for public health to redesign how it works with citizens and to move beyond a narrow view of volunteering that is concerned with directly improving physical and mental health, to support volunteering in a much more holistic way, such as engaging with tenants' and residents' groups or with volunteers involved in running sport, culture and leisure activities. In the medium term, through directly engaging with communities through HWBs, public health may even be able to help citizens bring greater local democratic accountability to one of the least accountable institutions in the country – the NHS itself. A recent report on health-improving councils by the New Local Government Network argues that 'although historically the public have had little input into what and how public health initiatives are rolled out, HWBs represent a unique opportunity to link up citizen representatives with decision makers' (Kuznetsova, 2012, p 61).

The transfer of responsibility for public health to local authorities follows growing interest shown by local authority councillors and officers in the health and well-being agenda, illustrated by local authority engagement in processes such as Local Area Agreements, programmes such as the Local Government Innovation and Development (LGID) Healthy Communities Programme, and the development of Joint Strategic Needs Assessments. Local authorities are themselves undergoing a period of transition from traditional service providers towards adopting a more enabling role with a focus on early intervention and place-based working at a neighbourhood level (Maginn, 2010; Michaelson, 2011). However, a Local Government Association report on well-being and the role of local government makes it clear that while councils welcome the new focus on well-being as a unifying and transformative agenda, there are significant concerns about their ability to deliver in the context of unprecedented cuts in funding (Michaelson, 2011).

At the same time as councils are taking on a greater role in health and well-being, there is a growing recognition that the approach that the Department of Health has been taking to address complex health challenges needs to be reconsidered in the light of significant criticism from the National Audit Office (2010) and the House of Commons Health Committee (2009) of the failure to make an impact on health inequalities. The last Labour government commissioned Sir Michael Marmot to undertake a strategic review of health inequalities in England. The subsequent report, *Fair society, healthy lives* (The Marmot Review, 2010a), which came out in 2010 under the current Coalition government, concludes that the fundamental drivers of inequalities in health are 'inequities in power, money and resources' (The Marmot Review, 2010a, p 16). The Marmot Review (2010a, p 30) recommends that one of the priority policy objectives should be to 'improve community capital and reduce social isolation across the gradient', noting that the 'extent of people's participation in their communities and the added control over their lives that this brings, has the potential to contribute to their psychosocial well–being and, as a result, to other health outcomes'. The review concludes by setting out an implementation framework to achieve reductions in health inequalities along the social gradient, stating that 'without citizen participation and community engagement fostered by public service organisations, it will be difficult to improve penetration of interventions and to impact on health inequalities' (The Marmot Review, 2010a, p 151). The Coalition government has indicated its support for the recommendations of The Marmot Review and most of them are reflected in its strategy for public health, *Healthy lives, healthy people* (Secretary of State for Health, 2010b). This seems somewhat perverse given current economic policies and the fact that inequality is growing faster than in any other developed country (Organisation for Economic Co-operation and Development, 2011); however, as discussed earlier in this chapter, the rhetoric of policy is all too frequently out of step with the actions governments take.

—

Rethinking the welfare state

Recent governments, whether Conservative, Labour or Coalition, have pursued welfare policies based on the belief that introducing market mechanisms into the public sector is the only way of increasing efficiency and making services affordable in the future. Marketisation is regarded as the only viable alternative to monolithic provision of welfare services by the state, the latter being viewed as having offered little in the way of choice, and having led to an inefficient public sector that serves the needs of its employees rather than the public. Those defending the welfare state point to its universality, reciprocity (Taylor-Goodby, 2009) and cost-effectiveness (Organisation for Economic Co-operation and Development, 2011). Boyle et al (2010a, p 3), however, argue that welfare services can create dependency, which not only disempowers, but tends also to 'create waste by failing to recognise service users' own strengths and assets, and to engender a culture of dependency that stimulates demand'.

Within mainstream discourse, these two models – statist or market-led provision – are frequently presented as the only alternatives, with the latter being seen as unquestionably the only way forward in times of economic restraint. The NEF, in its publication *Unintended Consequences*, debunks what it calls the 'myths' that lead to a 'narrow view of efficiency in public services' and questions the assumption that 'public services are best delivered through the market mechanism and the imitation of private sector incentive systems' (Ryan-Collins et al, 2007, p 11). So, if marketisation does not produce efficiency and state provision tends to disempower and create dependency rather than engagement, is there an alternative way forward? The NEF argues that the relationship between the state and its citizens needs to be reviewed not with the purpose of shrinking the state, but to create a different 'public benefit model' of public service delivery that offers 'new ways of conceptualising and measuring efficiency'. This model sees service users as having assets as well as needs and is based on co-production principles and on building sustainability at a local level (Ryan-Collins et al, 2007, p 15). These ideas are explored further in Chapter Twelve where a model of citizen-centred public health is proposed that would fit within a new conceptualisation of welfare services along the lines of the NEF's public benefit model.

Key points

- Volunteering is an act of citizenship and a component of a vibrant democracy. While much volunteering occurs independently of state activity, policy can stimulate and support citizen involvement.
- The concept of the Big Society is located within wider and enduring arguments for redefining the relationship between the state and its citizens, but, at the same time, symbolises an ideological drive for a smaller government.

- The importance of community engagement and volunteering for health and social care has been a consistent theme within Department of Health policy; however, the rhetoric has not always translated into mainstream policy reforms.
- Government support for strategies to increase social action and to tackle health inequalities are likely to be undermined by the impact of the retrenchment of public services, combined with any reduction in funding to the community and voluntary sector.

THREE

Lay health workers in practice

This chapter explores the recent history of lay people getting involved in health, starting with programmes established top-down by agencies external to the communities they serve – be they government, non-governmental organisations or charitable foundations – with a particular focus on community health workers. It then looks briefly at activities that have grown 'bottom-up' as a result of communities initiating action themselves. The aim of the chapter is to provide a context for considering lay health worker programmes designed to improve health in the English public health system and to reflect on learning from the successes and challenges elsewhere. It is acknowledged that many of the role titles found in the international literature often bear little relation to those used in current UK public health practice (see Chapter One). This is partly a reflection of public health policy, both current and past (see Chapter Two), and partly due to the differences in health systems across the world. The authors have tried to highlight parallel roles where appropriate.

The community health worker concept – history and practice

'Barefoot doctors' were introduced in China in the 1950s (Zhang and Unschuld, 2008), and some other countries had similar programmes from the 1950s and 1960s, but the term 'community health worker', and, indeed, 'primary health care', only came into general usage in the 1980s (Frankel and Doggett, 1992). This section traces a brief history of the development of the community health worker concept in the global South, and then the US, before tracing the history of similar programmes in the UK in the following section.

The concept of the community health worker was developed by the World Health Organization working closely with UNICEF (United Nations Children's Fund) over a period of several years in the 1970s (Walt, 1990; Frankel and Doggett, 1992). Health as an aspect of development had been neglected in the 1950s and 1960s when economic growth was seen as the primary, and often the only, goal of development and, furthermore, it was assumed that other benefits, such as health, would 'trickle down'. When it became clear that this was not happening, and, indeed, inequalities in general were widening, ideas on development started to change, with improvements in health seen as a necessary part of an integrated approach. A major concern was the lack of access to health services for rural populations in developing countries, together with the neglect of poor urban communities, and it was these concerns that underpinned the development of the concept of primary health care (World Health Organization, 1978). The dominance of the medical model and hospital-based care was increasingly challenged as often ineffective, culturally inappropriate and inaccessible to the poorest communities. The need to involve communities in the planning and provision of services was also recognised as essential to effective prevention and education for health (Rifkin, 2001).

All of these factors provided the context for a leading development agency, UNICEF, and the leading global agency for health, the World Health Organization, jointly to develop the community health worker concept, which became seen to enshrine all the principles adopted by the International Conference on Primary Health Care in Alma-Ata in 1978 (World Health Organization, 1978). *Health for all by the year 2000* (HFA 2000) (World Health Organization, 1981) had been launched at the Thirtieth World Assembly in the previous year, and the Declaration of Alma-Ata identified primary health care, and community health workers as a part of primary health care, as key to the delivery of HFA 2000. The definition of primary health care was broad to include the many factors that contribute to health, for example, agriculture, education and housing, as well as health services. The principles underpinning primary health care – a holistic approach to health, equity, community involvement, inter-sectoral collaboration and prevention – continue to be as relevant today as they were in 1978 (World Health Organization, 2008b).

Community health workers are lay people without clinical training who undertake basic health care and prevention activities, and, according to the World Health Organization, should be:

> members of the communities where they work, should be selected by the communities, should be answerable to the communities for their activities, should be supported by the health system but not necessarily a part of its organization, and have a shorter training than professional workers. (World Health Organization, 2007, p 1)

Following Alma-Ata, there was a rapid development of community health worker programmes in many countries, mainly in the global South. The community health worker programmes established across the world throughout the 1980s varied hugely; indeed, many did not use the term community health worker. Community health aide, family welfare educator, village health guide are but a few of the titles adopted (Lehmann and Sanders, 2007). Some programmes were set up following popular revolutions, for example, in Nicaragua (Petrack, 1984), some in the wake of independence, for example, in Tanzania (Heggenhougen et al, 1987), and were part of wider state efforts to improve the lot of the poorer sections of society. Some were generic, while others focused on one aspect of health, for example, malaria control or HIV/AIDS (Lehmann and Sanders, 2007).

Many differences between programmes are evident: some community health workers are paid, albeit a low wage; some receive honorariums; some are volunteers; some have five days' training, some three months'; some undertake a range of health care tasks, including prescribing drugs; some have a purely educational role.

Very few are selected by the communities where they work, although they are lay people, albeit generally with a somewhat higher level of education than the people they are working with (Lehmann and Sanders, 2007; Bhutta et al, 2010). More often than not, community health workers are part of the health system and as such are no longer truly part of the communities they work in. Walt (1990) concluded that they are usually 'just another pair of hands' at a health facility, which is not to say that what they are doing is not valuable, but their work is focused on individuals and their health rather than collective action to improve conditions or encouraging people to participate in improving their family's and community's health.

The 1980s, when community health worker programmes were growing rapidly, was a period of global economic downturn and many programmes were under-resourced and all too frequently expected to deliver too much in the absence of developments in primary health care and the rest of the health system. Frankel and Doggett (1992) commented that to blame community health workers for failing when programmes were often inadequately resourced, planned and supported is unfair. They point to the many successes of community health workers and argue that the debate needs to be about how to fulfil their potential, not whether they should exist. There is an inherent tension between the community health worker as an 'extender of health services' and as an 'agent of change' (Walt, 1990), and it was clearly unreasonable to expect, as was the case with some programmes, relatively untrained volunteers or low-paid workers to undertake the wide range of tasks given to them and thereby transform the health outcomes of very poor and marginalised communities. Notwithstanding these issues, many community health worker programmes have resulted in health benefits to the communities they serve, and positive health outcomes have been demonstrated from lay health worker interventions in primary and community health care (Lewin et al, 2005, 2006, 2010).

In recent years, there has been a resurgence of interest in community health workers and the World Health Organization promotes the mainstreaming of community health worker programmes as an essential part of primary health care (World Health Organization, 2007). The Pakistani and Brazilian case studies presented in Boxes 3.1 and 3.2, respectively, are examples of programmes that are being scaled up in an effort to address health challenges and inequalities.

Box 3.1: Pakistan's Lady Health Workers

The Pakistani government has invested millions of pounds in recruiting and training women recommended by their community to work as part of the health system to deliver a range of services to the community. They have three months classroom training and 12 months 'on the job' before taking responsibility for a community of, on average, 10,000 people. 'Lady Health Workers' receive a small allowance and medical supplies in order to provide treatment for common ailments as well as education in prevention. An external evaluation of the programme found that those communities with Lady Health Workers had markedly better health by a range of indicators than the control population. One example of international collaboration is where NHS Leeds is working in partnership with the Institute of Public Health in Lahore to promote smoke-free homes, with the Lady Health Workers promoting this message in Jia Bagga, a village near Lahore where the programme has been piloted.

Source: Department of Health (2010a).

Box 3.2: The Family Health Program in Brazil

The Family Health Program (Programa Sáuda da Família or PSF in Portuguese) can be considered the main government effort to improve primary health care in Brazil. The PSF provides a broad range of primary health care services delivered by a team composed of one physician, one nurse, a nurse assistant and (usually) four or more community health workers (community health agents). In some places, the team also includes dental and social work professionals. Each team is assigned to a geographical area and is then responsible for enrolling and monitoring the health status of the population living in that area, providing primary care services and making referrals to other levels of care as required. Each team is responsible for an average of 3,450 and a maximum of 4,500 people. Physicians and nurses typically deliver services at health facilities placed within the community, while community health agents provide health promotion and education services during household visits. As of 2004, the programme covered about 66 million people nationally, nearly 40% of the entire population. The results showed that PSF expansion, along with other socio-economic developments, were consistently associated with reductions in infant mortality. By early 2006, 60% of the population was looked after by 25,000 health teams.

Source: Adapted from Lehmann and Sanders (2007, p 9).

Where community health worker programmes have failed to deliver, it has generally been because of a lack of political commitment or support within the health system, poor-quality training, and inadequate supervision (Abbatt, 2005; Lehmann and Sanders, 2007). It is argued that effective scaling up is needed to address these shortcomings to build on the successes of many small programmes (Frankel and Doggett, 1992). For a summary of a review undertaken for the World Health Organization about what is known about community health workers and the factors that need to be taken into account to establish effective community health worker programmes (Lehmann and Sanders, 2007), see Box 3.3.

Box 3.3: Community health workers – key conclusions from an international review

- Community health workers [CHWs] can make a valuable contribution to community development and, more specifically, can improve access to and coverage of communities with basic health services.
- For CHWs to be able to make an effective contribution, they need to be carefully selected, appropriately trained and ... adequately and continuously supported.
- Large-scale CHW systems require substantial and reliable resources for training, management, supervision, and logistics.... Numerous programmes have failed in the past because of unrealistic expectations, poor planning and an underestimation of the effort and input required to make them work.
- Programmes are vulnerable unless they are driven, owned by and firmly embedded in communities themselves. Where this is not the case, they exist on the geographical and organizational periphery of the formal health system ... [and] are often fragile and unsustainable.
- The concept of community ownership and participation is often ill-conceived and poorly understood as a by-product of programmes initiated from the centre.
- Evidence suggests that CHW programmes thrive in mobilised communities, but struggle where they are given the responsibility of galvanising and mobilising communities.

Source: Lehmann and Sanders (2007, p 26).

Community health workers in the US

Although some examples can be found from the 1950s, community health worker activity in the US really started to grow in the 1960s when it was part of anti-poverty and, to a lesser extent, job-creation strategies (US Department of Health and Human Services et al, 2007). For example, a community health worker programme for Native American populations called the Community Representative Program originated from the Office of Economic Opportunity, but was later transferred to the Indian Health Service (Centers for Disease Control and Prevention, 2003). There was a steady growth in similar programmes aimed at poor communities through the 1970s and 1980s, which were often linked to research; hence the predominance of US studies in the published literature on community health workers (South et al, 2010b). A review of Lay Health Advisor programmes aimed at Hispanic/Latino communities (Rhodes et al, 2007) identified six primary roles:

- making contact with people and recruiting them to health programmes;
- health education and referral to health services;
- distribution of health information and resources, for example, condoms;
- being role models in the community;

- advocacy; and
- community research.

As programmes in the US developed, they started to standardise training and to link up and share good practice, and, from the early 1990s, the first state funding was put into community health worker programmes (US Department of Health and Human Services et al, 2007). Community health worker associations started to appear and a landmark study in 1994 described community health workers as 'integral members of the health care work force' (Witmer et al, 1995, p 1055). The first national study of community health workers, the National Community Health Adviser Study, was published in 1998 (Rosenthal et al, 1998). The American Public Health Association formed a Community Health Worker Special Interest Group in 2000, as community health worker practice and training became increasingly standardised and integrated into the health care system. Community health workers in the US continue to play an important role in promoting health and preventing ill health in the poorest communities in relation to a wide range of issues from cancer, tuberculosis and HIV/AIDS to child and maternal health (US Department of Health and Human Services et al, 2007). Although community health worker models are dominant, other approaches to involving lay people in public health are in evidence in North America, for example, Popular Opinion Leaders (Kelly et al, 1992; Kelly, 2004). Box 3.4 gives an example of volunteer involvement in a Canadian community-based cardiovascular prevention programme.

Box 3.4: Volunteers working in a clinical setting: the Cardiovascular Health Awareness Program in Ontario, Canada

The Cardiovascular Health Awareness Program (CHAP) is a community-based programme that recruits local people as volunteers to help undertake checks including blood pressure, particularly in people aged 65 and over, with the aim of reducing hypertension and, therefore, hospital admissions and mortality from heart disease and stroke. The main characteristics of the CHAP programme are as follows:

- CHAP invites older adults to their local pharmacy for a blood pressure reading, which is self-administered with the help of a volunteer. Advice is offered on healthy eating, physical activity and smoking cessation.
- CHAP participants can take home a copy of their results and give their permission to have this health information shared with their family physician and pharmacist. This allows physicians and pharmacists to follow-up with their patients if required.
- A randomised control trial was conducted, the CHAP programme being implemented in 20 communities of 10,000–60,000 people with 19 comparable communities acting as controls.
- Over the trial period, 577 volunteers conducted 27,358 risk assessments with 15,889 participants (some were invited back for further blood pressure monitoring). Results

> show a reduction in hospital admissions for cardiovascular disease at a population level in the intervention communities.
>
> - The full support of local physicians and pharmacies, together with a standardised implementation package led from the centre, were key elements to the successful roll-out of the programme.
> - Recruitment of volunteers was straightforward and effective training and support was important. Volunteers were key to 'spreading the word' and ensuring very good uptake (some sessions had to be extended to cope with the numbers) as well as providing the one-to-one support participants needed.
> - As of autumn 2009, the CHAP programme was still ongoing in 16 communities and results from spring 2008 showed that 3,652 participants had been screened by 137 volunteers. Of the 9.4% of participants with high blood pressure readings, 55.0% were diagnosed with hypertension, 15.7% with diabetes and 42.8% with high cholesterol.
>
> *Sources:* Carter et al (2009), Kaczorowski et al (2011) and CHAP (2009).

Lay health workers in the UK

The UK has not developed formal community health worker programmes as in the US and countries in the global South. However, as health care costs have continued to spiral, there has been an increasing emphasis on self-care, patient involvement and reducing the factors that place people at risk of ill health (Wanless, 2004; Imison et al, 2011). This has led to the establishment of some national programmes in recent years, such as Walking for Health (described in Chapter Six), the Expert Patients Programme, community health champions and the Health Trainer Programme (described later in the chapter). In addition, there are many initiatives outside the health field that are helping to improve health and well-being. One example is Home-Start, which, through a network of nearly 16,000 trained parent volunteers, supports parents who are struggling to cope for a whole variety of reasons, for example, postnatal illness, disability, bereavement, the illness of a parent or child, or social isolation (Home-Start, no date).

The Expert Patient Programme

The Expert Patient Programme was launched in 2001 by the Department of Health and consists of lay-led programmes in self-management for people with long-term conditions. At the core of the Expert Patient Programme is a six-week (one session per week) course, adapted from the Chronic Disease Self Management Programme in the US, delivered by lay people who have a long-term condition to their peers. The course is generic (not condition-specific) and delivery follows a standard model (Expert Patients Programme, 2011).

An evaluation of the Expert Patient Programme, which included a randomised control trial involving 629 participants, was carried out by the National Primary

Care Research and Development Centre (Rogers et al, 2006). Overall, the evaluation found that the programme did increase self-efficacy by a moderate amount and that participants particularly enjoyed the group experience. Rogers et al (2006, p ii) concluded that the 'programme is likely to be cost effective because there was an overall reduction in service utilisation which offset the costs of the intervention'. They did, however, note that participants tended to be white, middle class, well educated and already committed to self-managing. They also noted that it was proving difficult to embed the programme as health professionals were proving slow to get on board, in part because of the generic nature of the course. While volunteer tutors were very committed, the lack of specific training in facilitation, plus the rather rigid, generic nature of the programme, meant that it was not always as useful to participants as it could have been (Rogers et al, 2006).

In 2007, the Expert Patient Programme Community Interest Company (EPP CIC) was established as a not-for-profit social enterprise to continue the roll-out of the programme. A mixture of volunteers, contracted staff and bank staff are currently used to deliver its range of services. In October 2010, courses were commissioned by over 50% of Primary Care Trusts in England and across all local health boards in Wales, and are a key part of Scottish heath policy. Over 100,000 people have used Expert Patients Programme services and over 2,000 volunteer lay tutors have been trained nationwide (Expert Patients Programme, 2011).

Health trainers

Since 2004, the Department of Health has been supporting the roll-out of health trainer programmes across England (Department of Health, 2005a). Health trainers are the first public health workforce in the country to be recruited from communities with the poorest health, with the explicit purpose of addressing inequalities. They are non-clinical workers who receive training to engage target communities and then provide one-to-one support for people who want to make a change to improve their health and connect them into activities in their local area that will help them maintain those changes. Most health trainers are paid workers, usually on a salaried basis but sometimes sessionally. By February 2010, nearly 90% of Primary Care Trusts had set up a health trainer service (Department of Health, 2010b). These vary in size, focus and location according to local priorities; some health trainers are working in GP practices as part of primary care teams, others are community-based and work to engage those often described as 'hard to reach' (Yorkshire and Humber Regional Health Trainer Hub, 2011). Health trainers are increasingly supported by health trainer champions, who are volunteers who have a short training programme to enable them to support health trainers through outreach work (Department of Health, 2008a). Health trainer champions have been introduced into offender settings, for example, half of prisons in Yorkshire and Humber now have trained prisoners to support other inmates to adopt healthier lifestyles (Health Trainers England, no date).

Health trainers can be described as a type of community health worker as they work between health services and local communities, supporting people from their own or similar communities (South et al, 2007). The White Paper *Choosing health*, where the role was first introduced, saw this as signalling a shift from 'advice from on high to support from next door' (Department of Health, 2004, p 106). (For a case story of a health trainer supporting a client, see Box 3.5.) Much of what has been learnt about how to run an effective health trainer programme mirrors the conclusions of the international review of community health worker programmes (see Box 3.4). In particular, recruiting from communities, working collaboratively with community and health care organisations, a standardised training programme with regular updates, frequent supervision, appropriate protocols and practice guidance, proper monitoring, and adequate resources to do the role are all key elements. Furthermore, health trainers need time to engage with people effectively and access to other community activities that can provide clients with the ongoing social support often needed to maintain changes in lifestyle.

Box 3.5: A case study of health trainer support for a client newly diagnosed with diabetes

Mark (not his real name) was 66 years old, living in a disadvantaged neighbourhood on the east coast of England, who was referred to the health trainer service by a local charity. He had recently been diagnosed with diabetes and also had heart problems. He lived on his own and he wanted to be more active and to understand more about healthy eating in order to control his diabetes.

The health trainer advised Mark to make an appointment to see the diabetic nurse specialist and Mark asked the health trainer to accompany him as he "could not take in the information they had told him before". The health trainer explained what happened next:

> "When we came out [of the appointment], I was able to go through what had been said to him and he had only retained a small amount, so we went to the local library and talked it through. The next time we met, we went to the local supermarket and looked at the food labels and I showed him different alternatives to eat and drink and introduced him to other foods, especially ones with low sugar and fat.... Finding out some of what he'd done in the past was very useful, he'd really enjoyed hiking, it had been a way for him to reduce stress. So I introduced him to a small walking group."

The result was that Mark began losing weight slowly, with additional support from the health trainer to keep his motivation high. He started walking regularly and the health trainer also asked his GP for exercise referral, so he was able to join the gym. The health trainer stated:

> "Mark's diet has much improved and he is slowly changing his lifestyle. I only met with Mark five times, but I have a chat with him by phone once a week and keep encouraging him in the right direction.... Mark lacked confidence in most areas of his life and I think working

---

> with a health trainer he found someone he could talk to and did not feel embarrassed to ask the simplest question. I also learnt how a little support can go a long way.'"

Source: Adapted from White and South (2012, p 28).

Volunteering for health and community health champions

In 2009/10, 25% of people in England had participated in formal volunteering in the past month, and 40% in the past 12 months. Furthermore, 29% of people said they had volunteered informally at least once in the last month, rising to over 50% in the last 12 months (Department for Communities and Local Government, 2011). While these figures show high levels of volunteering in the general population, the number of people who had volunteered informally had declined quite markedly from previous years (Department for Communities and Local Government, 2011). In health and social care, volunteers undertake a range of roles, including: helping to organise an event; providing transport; giving information; counselling; visiting or befriending service users; and mentoring (Hawkins and Restall, 2006). Surveys by Volunteering England have found that volunteering is good for the health of both volunteers and those they are helping; indeed, many volunteers are former service users who want to 'give something back' (Teasdale, 2008, p 3).

There is no national overview of the myriad ways in which volunteers are helping people to improve their health, but the People in Public Health study was able to form a picture of the range and variety of lay activity. Much of this occurs outside of public health structures but benefits health, for example, the volunteer effort that keeps sports clubs going and enables thousands of young people in particular to participate in regular physical activity. Most programmes that involve volunteers are locally, rather than nationally, coordinated, some at a neighbourhood level. Often, these are very informal, but many formal public health programmes also engage volunteers. For example, in 2007, the Bradford & Airedale Teaching Primary Care Trust supported volunteers working, among other things, as breastfeeding peer supporters, stop smoking service community advisers, walk leaders and buddies for people with HIV/AIDS, and, in addition, provided free, accredited training for people to become community health activists (South et al, 2010b, p 14).

The concept of 'community health champions' – volunteers who improve health in a wide variety of ways using an empowerment approach to engage communities experiencing the poorest health – has emerged onto the public health agenda in recent years (Secretary of State for Health, 2010b). Altogether Better, which originated in Yorkshire and Humber and was funded through the Big Lottery well-being fund, has spearheaded the development of a community health champion model (Altogether Better, no date). Altogether Better, working through Primary Care Trusts, local government and voluntary groups, uses an empowerment approach that seeks to equip health champions with the knowledge, confidence

Figure 2.1: The Altogether Better empowerment model

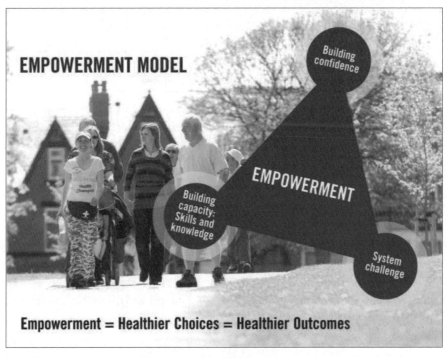

Source: Altogether Better Regional Programme Team (2009).

and skills to make a difference in their communities, but with the ultimate aim of producing 'system challenge' as participants become more empowered. Altogether Better projects have been successful in recruiting people from a range of different communities, who then receive training and support from the projects to enable them to become community health champions and carry out voluntary activities in neighbourhoods and workplaces (Altogether Better, 2010). Since the programme was established in 2008, over 15,000 health champions have been recruited and they have connected with a further 90,000 people. Some health champions are now working within primary care, for example, a pilot project is involving health champions and health trainers working as part of care pathways for people with diabetes (see Chapter Ten) (Altogether Better, no date).

Community action – volunteering from the bottom up

In the 1960s and 1970s, some people in both the developing and developed world started to become active in their own health, often as part of a wider social movement like the women's movement and movements that organised to challenge medical models by creating alternative social models of disability and mental illness. Health social movements generally fall into one of three categories: those challenging lack of access to health; those representing a particular constituency, for example, related to sexuality, ethnicity or gender; and those representing the interests of people with a particular health condition or disability (Brown and Zavestoski, 2005). All seek to challenge the system and, to a greater or lesser extent, the existing power structures within it. For example, the women's health movement has sought to challenge the domination of the medical model and professional, male definitions of female health. The book *Our bodies, ourselves* (Phillips and Rakusen, 1978), which championed a woman's right to be respected as an expert in her own health, has continued to be popular since it was first published in the US in 1971 and in the UK in 1978. The book arose from the activities of the Boston Women's Health Collective in the US, where women who were active as volunteers in promoting women's health researched and wrote the book together.

People with a disability have also become increasingly active in challenging medical models of disability over the last 40 years with the emergence of a wide range of organisations controlled and run by disabled people, which Oliver (1997) argues constitute a social movement when taken together. The number of disability-related support services controlled and run by disabled people themselves has increased significantly in the UK and internationally over the last few decades (Barnes and Mercer, 2006), and the involvement of people with a disability or mental illness in service provision and delivery has become a key priority for many governments. However, Cowden and Singh (2007) argue that in the UK, because the move towards greater involvement of users has taken place within a context of increasing regulation, this has not led to true engagement in fully integrated services.

Linked to health and disability social movements, through the 1980s, community development projects, which sought to actively engage people in determining their own priorities and how to address them, broadened to include an explicit focus on health (Tones and Tilford, 2001). Many community health initiatives developed, sometimes as part of bigger health, community and/or regeneration programmes, sometimes formed 'bottom up' by communities themselves (Smithies and Webster, 1998; Amos, 2002). Many of these initiatives were relatively short-lived, but some are still active and engage community members in a variety of projects to improve their health.

In Scotland, the Community Health Exchange provides a support network for community health projects (Community Health Exchange, no date). The Exchange seeks to influence policy, to provide information and establish networks so that projects can support each other, and to develop practice by:

- promoting opportunities to enhance practice in community development approaches to health improvement;
- promoting community-led health research and supporting communities to undertake their own research and take forward findings;

- building the capacity of community members to address and take action on their priority health issues through participation in the 'Health Issues in the Community' training initiative; and
- supporting tutors to deliver and evaluate the 'Health Issues in the Community' training initiative (Community Health Exchange, no date).

Some health movements continue to be an integral part of the struggles of disempowered communities. One striking example is the Zapatista movement in Mexico, which has set up an alternative health system built and run by volunteers from the indigenous communities it serves (see Box 3.6). The Zapatista health clinics are an illustration of the principles of Alma–Ata in action, as they provide accessible and culturally appropriate primary health care and preventive services for the local population, and their health workers are selected and supported by the communities they serve, as originally proposed by the World Health Organization (World Health Organization, 1987, 2007).

Box 3.6: Creating an alternative health system: the Zapatistas in Mexico

The Zapatistas have continued to struggle for social and economic change in Mexico for over 100 years. One of the gains made since the Zapatista uprising of 1994 has been the creation of a partially liberated zone of thousands of square kilometres. Within this zone, thousands of Zapatista communities have carried out a long-running experiment in self-management. Sometimes, this has been on land they have occupied, but more often, it is on new land cleared from the Lacanodon jungle in the decades before 1994.

The importance of this zone is that it provides a space in which the methods of self-determination advocated by the Zapatistas are being put into practice. This is in the most difficult circumstances, for even without the army and paramilitary presence, the extreme poverty, lack of education and infrastructure would present formidable barriers. The areas the Zapatistas operate in are rural and extremely poor. Small communities of a dozen to over 100 families are typical, forced to live off the land without the benefit of modern agricultural machinery.

Within the autonomous zone, indigenous communities have created their own health service, because the government system has proved expensive, discriminatory and inadequate. The smaller villages have a 'health house' where a trained volunteer health promoter can provide limited advice and care. Then there are larger clinics that can provide treatment for the many diseases common in the area and reproductive care. They are staffed by more experienced health workers, chosen by their peers, who do not receive a salary but are provided with shelter and food by the community. The clinics themselves were built by volunteer labour with support from international solidarity movements. They exist despite, and without the

---

support of, the Mexican authorities and manage to provide basic primary health care that is free and culturally appropriate.

Sources: Adapted from Edinburgh Chiapas Solidarity Group (2011), Irish Mexico Group (2001), Davies (2009) and Kozart (2007).

Conclusion

This chapter has presented a brief historical overview of how lay people have engaged, and continue to engage, in health. The picture is a very varied and complex one, with interventions varying from top–down initiatives to train and deploy a community workforce to meet deficiencies in the existing health system, through to social movements that aim to challenge existing power structures that perpetuate poor health and inequalities. This overview provides a context for the theme of the book to explore the role of lay people in promoting their own health. At times, this can present challenges to established systems, as can participatory approaches in general, particularly within professionally dominated health systems. Lay health workers, in both paid and voluntary roles, are being incorporated into the workforce structure of the public health system in England, but, arguably, this does not detract from the rights of people to challenge through collective action where the system does not meet their needs.

Key points

- There is a long history of community health worker programmes in the global South and in North America. The field of practice is very diverse, with community health workers involved in delivering primary health care and/or health promotion across a range of health issues and population groups.
- Much of what has been learned about community health worker programmes, notably the need for professional support from within the health system and the importance of community participation and ownership, has relevance for UK public health.
- Consideration of lay health worker roles needs to take account of social movements for health where people take action on health based on community not professional priorities.
- In England, there are many people volunteering in health and social care, and, in addition, national initiatives that recruit and support lay health workers in providing peer support and engaging people in health activity are adding to public health capacity.

FOUR

Benefits and value

This chapter looks at the main justifications for involving members of the public in delivering public health programmes. It draws on findings from the People in Public Health study to present some core reasons why services might wish to involve members of the public (South et al, 2010b). Indeed, there was remarkable consistency around these reasons in the different elements of the study. Some of the emerging themes discussed here will be explored in more depth in the case studies of public health projects in Chapters Six to Nine, but this chapter provides an overview of the main arguments around benefits and value, and also briefly discusses drawbacks. In addition, the issue of the evidence base is tackled by critically examining categorisations of outcomes, as well as economic and moral arguments.

Six key reasons for engaging members of the public in programme delivery

1. To provide an essential bridging function reducing barriers between services and communities, particularly where groups are at risk of social exclusion

The potential for members of the public to act as bridges, improving the connections between health services and communities, forms a strong justification, particularly where health inequalities are present due to poverty or other forms of disadvantage. Bridging is a dominant theme in the case studies in Chapters Six to Nine. In many of the US models, such as Lay Health Advisors, involving lay people in programme delivery is considered a vital strategy for addressing health disparities in underserved and low-income communities, mostly African-American and Hispanic/Latino (Jackson and Parks, 1997; Bailey et al, 2005; Perez-Escamilla et al, 2008; Fleury et al, 2009). Lay health workers are typically engaged in a range of activities, including health education, outreach, cultural mediation, advocacy, social support and signposting to other services within their communities (Swider, 2002; Andrews et al, 2004; Rhodes et al, 2007). The assumptions are that lay health workers, recruited from local communities, will bring local knowledge and understanding of community norms, cultural competence and access to social networks, and will speak the same language (McQuiston and Uribe, 2001; Rhodes et al, 2007). In some models, there is an explicit aim to identify through community networks what are called 'natural helpers' in those communities, who are trusted by community members (Watkins et al, 1994; Jackson and Parks, 1997). The American Association of Diabetes Educators (2003, p 821) describes community health workers as:

uniquely skilled to serve as bridges between community members and healthcare services because they live in the communities in which they work, understand what is meaningful, and communicate in the language of the people in their communities. They know the cultural buffers, such as cultural identity, spiritual coping, and traditional health practices that can help community members cope with stress and promote positive health outcomes. A critical asset of programmes that engage community health workers is that they build on already existing community network ties that contribute to the acceptance and sustainability of effective community programs.

Bringing lay people with local and experiential knowledge into programme delivery has a number of advantages for public health and health care services. Witmer et al (1995) argue that community health workers can: (1) increase access to care; (2) improve the quality of care; (3) reduce the cost of care; and (4) make a broader social contribution by enabling individual and community empowerment. For communities, access to health and welfare services can be improved by lay health workers communicating information about services and available resources, being role models, and helping people navigate their way through services. This can be a vital role where there are barriers because of language, or where social exclusion and stigmatisation exists; for example, link workers from minority ethnic communities work in NHS primary care services to help service users get access to services, offering interpretation as needed (Levenson and Gillam, 1998). Brownstein et al (2007), reporting on community health worker interventions for people with hypertension mostly from African–American and other minority ethnic populations, identified lay health worker roles such as acting as mediators between clients and health and social care systems and ensuring that clients received services necessary for hypertension control, including assistance with insurance matters, referrals and arranging for transport to appointments. A UK example of this type of approach is the Connected Care navigators developed by Turning Point (2010).

Improved connections between services and communities can help health professionals gain better access to a population that is deemed 'hard-to-reach' and translate messages into the social context of the community (Kennedy et al, 2008a). The concept of social networks is important here as lay health workers will normally have good access to the community and their messages will have credibility (McQuiston and Uribe, 2001; Taylor et al, 2001). In some programmes, lay health workers act as conduits between the community and the service and allow programmes to respond flexibly to changing community needs (Witmer et al, 1995).

Bridging is dependent on a set of interrelationships between professionals and lay workers and between lay workers and communities (South et al, 2012). The implications are that lay health workers need to be accepted and trusted by professionals, but, perhaps more critically, need to remain oriented to their community and reflect the characteristics of that community (Eng et al, 1997). The effectiveness of these approaches is likely to be reduced where lay health workers become professionalised and incorporated into the workforce (Jackson and Parks, 1997; Love et al, 2004), although individual lay health workers should clearly be enabled to progress.

2. To reduce communication barriers as lay workers have the potential to reach some communities that professionals cannot

Lay involvement is often sought in public health programmes because of lay health workers' cultural competence within specific contexts and their ability to communicate effectively with target communities (McQuiston and Uribe, 2001). This means that health messages can be successfully passed on to audiences that might otherwise face barriers to receiving or understanding that information. This is not to imply that communication is necessarily all about professional messages, the peer-led, client-centred model of health trainers shows how peer-based approaches can be about communication as dialogue (White and Kinsella, 2011; White et al, 2011). Shiner (1999) discusses how peer education is a naturally occurring activity, and therefore peer education projects can be about giving validity to lay experience and personal development with the aim of empowering people from disadvantaged groups who are able to relate to members of their communities. Coufopoulos et al (2010) found that community food workers, whose role was to communicate health messages and develop skills around cooking, eating and shopping, were using very flexible, informal client-centred strategies in working with communities.

Frankham (1998, p 179) reports that peer education has been characterised as 'a radical approach with clear cut benefits for reaching constituencies who have been impervious to personal and social education of more "traditional" forms'. Although Frankham and other commentators have questioned the validity of peer education interventions (see Kelly, 2004), involving peers in public health programmes is, nonetheless, justified on the basis of better reach, communication, acceptability and cultural sensitivity (Hart, 1998; Parkin and McKeganey, 2000; Taylor et al, 2001). Thus, peer-based approaches are particularly appropriate where groups are marginalised, such as drug users or people who are homeless (Hunter and Power, 2002), where there is a need to reduce stigma, as with sexual health interventions around HIV/AIDS (Stevens, 1994; Fernandez et al, 2003), or where the cultural context presents unique challenges, for example, in prisons (Collica, 2002; Ross et al, 2006). In some contexts, lay knowledge of neighbourhoods and social networks allows a programme to extend reach (Chiu and West, 2007), and addresses issues of access, for example, increasing the reach of screening programmes (Lam et al, 2003).

The concept of a peer or a peer group and its importance in health promotion is critical here. A peer is defined as someone of the same ability, standing or status (Dennis, 2003); in other words, someone who is an equal, not someone who is in the position of authority and power over the group they wish to influence. A recent report entitled 'Mindspace' examined how policy might 'nudge' people into different, more positive behaviours and summarised behavioural influences (Dolan et al, 2010, p 8):

- we are influenced by who communicates information;
- we are strongly influenced by what others do;
- we 'go with the flow' of pre-set options;
- our attention is drawn to what is novel and seems relevant to us;
- our acts are often influenced by subconscious cues;
- our emotional associations can powerfully shape our actions;
- we seek to be consistent with our public promises and reciprocate acts; and
- we act in ways that make us feel better about ourselves.

It is important to understand the basis of peer identity (Shiner, 1999). People can share similar attributes, like age or gender, or a have shared identity, for example, being a member of a faith community, or can share a common experience, like having diabetes. Such community identities are evidently dependent on context and can be expected to be fluid. Lay health workers are not always peers in the true sense of the word, as 'natural helpers' and 'community leaders' can have very different attributes from the community of interest (Taylor et al, 2001; Foster-Fishman et al, 2009), yet still offer access into the community.

3. To provide peer support to other community members to help them achieve better health

The importance of social support on health is well documented (Cooper et al, 1999; Friedli, 2009; Veenstra, 2000; Wilkinson and Marmot, 2003). Peer support is the more specific support provided and received by those who share similar attributes or types of experience. Dennis (2003) provides a concept analysis of peer support in health care contexts, which shows that peer support is a broad concept that can be applied in different settings, in response to different stressors and through different nodes of interaction, such as one to one or in groups. Dennis argues that peer support can work in three ways, through:

1. Direct effects – such as enhancing social relationships, facilitating access to health resources, and reducing isolation.
2. Buffering effects – protecting individuals from stressful events or promoting coping skills.
3. Mediating effect – modifying self-efficacy through positive encouragement and providing role models.

The value of peer support as a justification for involving members of the public can be considered on a number of levels. Volunteering as an activity has its roots in mutualism and philanthropy (Hardill et al, 2007) and peer support is a core element in much volunteering activity (Neuberger, 2008). While not all volunteers in health and health care are 'peers' in the true sense of the word, many provide an alternative (lay) source of support to professional care, which is often valued by those receiving services (Faulkner, 2005). The report *Seeing is believing* (Volunteering England, no date) points out that volunteering can impact on the quality of services by: (1) improving accessibility, as people may accept services more readily from a volunteer; (2) making a more diverse service; (3) providing a feedback mechanism; and (4) providing additional support.

Involving members of the public in the delivery of public health programmes will almost inevitably introduce an element of peer support, whatever the primary focus of the intervention. The rationale is that the inclusion of a lay element will mitigate some of the barriers to seeking professional advice or assistance, as well as promoting engagement in healthy activities. The value of the 'comfort factor', that is, seeing a friendly face, feeling welcomed and lowering levels of anxiety, may be a critical factor (Flax and Earp, 1999). Service users in the People in Public Health study spoke of the value they placed on the care and support they received (see Chapter Five). Often, this support, whether emotional, practical or cultural, was the critical factor in participation, and, moreover, service users supported other group participants (South et al, 2012). Peer support can be mutually beneficial both to those who help and to those who receive help; psychosocial benefits have been reported for volunteers engaged in peer support (Casiday et al, 2008).

A further justification relates to peer support as a mechanism for promoting health where the various effects of peer support are harnessed to achieve health goals. Examples include breastfeeding peer support (Dennis, 2002; Watt et al, 2006) and listening schemes in prisons (Farrant and Levenson, 2002). Britton et al (2006) describe the role of breastfeeding peer supporters as including forming relationships with mothers, sharing experiences and information, providing social support, giving time, and being a role model. Another example can be found with 'Fag Ends', a lay-led community-based smoking cessation service, where a process evaluation showed that community members using the service valued the mutual support – 'the sense that someone understands what you are going through' (Springett et al, 2007, p 252) – that they received from the group sessions as well as from the lay smoking cessation advisors.

4. To increase service capacity by having a 'community workforce' as well as a professional workforce

Involving lay people in programme delivery can increase the capacity of services to meet health needs through increasing the number of people available who can deliver public health or health care. This can work at a basic level by members of the public providing 'an extra pair of hands', which enables public health programmes to achieve coverage and scale. The increase in service capacity can be a critical factor. It is difficult to imagine that Walking for Health, the national health walks programme, would have achieved its activity levels without the contribution of the 11,000 plus walk leaders, many of whom are volunteers (Natural England, 2011a).

Constraints on professional time have been cited as a motivation for citizen involvement in service delivery, as having a 'lay workforce' can free up professionals to focus on areas of work that require their high-level skills. Kennedy et al (2008b) see this as a major driver in the development of the lay food and health worker role. A further example of this rationale can be found in the community-based childhood obesity programme 'Watch-It', where lay health workers are trained to support young people and families to achieve weight loss (Rudolf et al, 2006). In establishing the service, it was recognised that there were insufficient professional dieticians to deliver the level of personal support needed and the programme has since proved a relatively low-cost intervention that is valued by families and places little pressure on existing NHS services (see the case study in South and Sahota, 2010).

Notwithstanding debates about how a 'workforce' is defined and whether lay engagement can be considered as part of workforce development, increasing workforce capacity is a powerful motivation in some contexts. In the global South, recruiting and training community health workers is an important strategy to address capacity issues when health systems are under-resourced and there are insufficient health professionals (Hongoro and McPake, 2004; see also Chapter Three). A Department for International Development (DFID) report argues for the scaling up of community health worker programmes on the basis that community health workers have a shorter and less costly training than clinical staff, can communicate more effectively with local communities, and can increase the coverage of primary health care, particularly in rural areas (Abbatt, 2005).

While the issue of capacity has evidently been a driver in less economically developed countries, the extent to which these arguments apply in the English public health system can be questioned. While there may be variations in the coverage of services, the population has universal access to health care that is free at the point of delivery. Derek Wanless, a prominent banker, undertook wide-ranging reviews for the HM Treasury, first of the NHS (Wanless, 2002) and later of public health (Wanless, 2004). The reviews involved modelling different futures in relation to both supply and demand and his conclusions were that, without greater public engagement in health, demand would outstrip supply, whereas a 'fully engaged scenario' with high levels of public engagement in health would be the optimum scenario, resulting in lower levels of public expenditure and better health outcomes.

Citizen involvement can be justified in terms of mobilising community resources to support good health. Here, the justification concerns the ability and capacity of people to determine their own priorities and to develop solutions to problems in line with community development principles (Amos, 2002; Ledwith, 2005). This book does not discuss community development approaches in any depth; however, there are evident areas of overlap between community development and enabling people to take on public health roles. Chapter Three provides some examples of lay health workers in the context of social movements. The key issue is one of purpose with a distinction made between instrumental and empowerment models:

> Communities have a wealth of untapped resources and energy that can be harnessed and mobilized through community participation, using a range of practical techniques that can engage people and, where appropriate, train and employ them in community development work. There is a clear tension here between mobilizing resources in a way that empowers communities and mobilizing to reduce the cost of providing services. (World Health Organization, 2002, p 13)

5. To offer an opportunity for people to gain directly in terms of increased confidence, health literacy, self-fulfilment, social contact, skills and employability

The benefits of the act of volunteering are well versed in the literature on volunteering. It can be rewarding, lead to personal fulfilment, provide social contact and friendships (Dingle and Heath, 2001; Borgonovi, 2008; Neuberger, 2008). Volunteers chose to volunteer for a variety of reasons, including altruistic reasons, wanting to keep busy and because of a personal turning point (Brooks, 2002), but, regardless of motivation, there is evidence that the act of volunteering is beneficial for both mental and physical health (Casiday et al, 2008). Wilson (2000, p 232) cautions that there may be some self-selection, as healthy people may be more likely to volunteer; however, he goes on to say that 'good health is preserved by volunteering; it keeps healthy volunteers healthy'. In contrast to this view on self-selection, the People in Public Health study found many examples of people who had come into volunteering with health conditions or because of their experience as a service user. More often, these people reported that their involvement had a positive impact on them, leading to improved quality of life and functioning, or adoption of more healthy lifestyles (see Chapter Five).

The personal impact of involvement should be taken into account as part of the 'package' of citizen involvement and this aspect may represent a major motivation for programmes, particularly those focused on personal development and empowerment (Shiner, 1999), such as the Community Health Educators programme discussed in Chapter Eight. There are many examples of reported benefits for those engaged in lay health worker and other volunteer roles, including improvements in self-esteem and self-efficacy, social support, acquiring knowledge and skills, and giving a sense of purpose (Hainsworth and Barlow, 2003; Attree, 2004; Visram and Drinkwater, 2005; Curtis et al, 2007). Additionally, one of the themes that emerged from the expert hearings is the enjoyment and fun that people often experience in these roles (South et al, 2010b).

Participation can provide a springboard for individuals to pursue further training or education and to gain valuable life skills as well as increase employability. While there has been an emphasis in government policy on the value of volunteering as a step to employment (Cabinet Office, 2010), it should be noted that a 2008 survey commissioned by the Cabinet Office revealed that over half of people volunteer for altruistic reasons to help people, with only 7% doing it to help their career (Low et al, 2008, p 34). Nonetheless, for some individuals, participation does act as a route to gaining subsequent employment (Attree, 2004; Love et al, 2004; Neuberger, 2008). This notion of a skills escalator that allows people from disadvantaged communities to enter the public health workforce was one of the primary drivers for the introduction of the Health Trainer Programme (Department of Health, no date, 2004). With peer-based approaches in prison settings, there is evidence that peer helpers may reintegrate successfully into the community through finding paid employment (Ross et al, 2006) and have an increased propensity to embrace law-abiding values (Devilly et al, 2005).

6. To open up a conduit so that information can be cascaded through social networks and community knowledge can be fed back up to inform strategic planning and service delivery

Justifications for citizen involvement in programme delivery relate to more generic rationales for community participation as a key process underpinning a more healthy and equitable society (World Health Organization, 2002). The National Institute for Health and Clinical Excellence (NICE) guidance on community engagement proposes that higher levels of involvement will lead to more health outcomes in part through the utilisation of experiential knowledge leading to improved services (National Institute for Health and Clinical Excellence, 2008, p 7). Lay health workers bring experiential knowledge into services and, as discussed earlier, can enhance communication through community networks (Witmer et al, 1995). Lay knowledge is distinctive (El Ansari et al, 2002) and, moreover, may fundamentally challenge expert knowledge, leading to better explanations of health inequalities (Popay et al, 1998). Gaining community intelligence on community needs can help services develop more citizen-centred services that are better placed to meet health needs. As the case studies in Chapters Six to Nine show, local knowledge is important for the effective delivery of public health programmes.

Notwithstanding that community engagement needs to be at many levels in the public health system (National Institute for Health and Clinical Excellence, 2008), and to include representative as well as consultative mechanisms, citizen involvement in service delivery can provide a means to garner community views and to break down the barriers between services and communities so that meaningful dialogue can take place. One example of this is the North Carolina Breast Cancer Screening Program (Altpeter et al, 1998), where there were three elements: 'OutReach' through a volunteer network of older African-American women; 'Access' to reduce barriers to services; and 'InReach' to increase community influence in service planning. Professional community workers acted as coaches and provided opportunities for training and skills development in order to support community members' efforts at organising themselves and participating in service planning.

Instrumental approaches to citizen involvement are sometimes contrasted to the constitutive value of participation, as discussed later in this chapter. Rogers and Robinson (2004, p 9), for example, distinguish between community engagement as a means to 'ensure that services are more responsive and sensitive to the needs of those they are meant to serve' and the goal of civic renewal, where engaging communities in 'governing and running public services can foster trust, generate networks, teach skills and empower those who are engaged'. Evidence from public health practice suggests that both goals can coexist; nonetheless, at the expert hearings, which were conducted as part of the People in Public Health study (see Appendix), one expert witness cautioned:

> "If we start off with the philosophy that having lay people involved is about a more efficient way of delivering health services we've actually lost the plot.... I think it is actually about citizenship in a very broad way. It's about people being involved and taking a place in shaping what happens for themselves, for their families and their communities." (Expert hearing 2)

Drawbacks

Any discussion of the disadvantages of citizen involvement in the delivery of public health programmes must first acknowledge the absence of the topic from the research literature. There is discussion of rationales, of roles, of barriers to involvement from both professional and lay perspectives, but very little on the potential or actual drawbacks. Some drawbacks were identified in the People in Public Health case studies, but these were not dominant themes compared to the extensive discussion of benefits arising from involving members of the public. Drawbacks identified included:

- lay health workers lacking the knowledge base of professionals;
- lay health workers not being under professional control;
- the risk of lay health workers giving out incorrect information;
- the reliability of volunteers compared to paid staff, as they were not under the same obligations to the service; and
- the turnover of volunteers taking up project resources.

There is some discussion of risk in the volunteering literature. The risks to organisations and their service users from involving volunteers include: service users being misleading or giving incorrect advice; volunteers not adhering to role boundaries; breaches in confidentiality; and volunteers not being able to deal with emotional issues arising from the role (Faulkner, 2005; Gaskin, 2006a). These issues can be addressed by good volunteer management, including adequate training and supervision (Gaskin, 2006b; Hawkins and Restall, 2006). There can also be risks to the lay health worker when working in outreach services in high-risk contexts, for example, HIV-prevention outreach work with intravenous drug users (Dickson-Gomez et al, 2003), but these are the same risks faced by all working is those contexts.

Understanding outcomes

The implications of the various rationales for citizen involvement in programme delivery are that involvement will lead to positive changes in health and the determinants of health. This in turn raises the issue of effectiveness. In order to answer that question, there needs to be consideration of what is meant by success, a topic that is discussed further in Chapter Eleven. The People in Public Health study, although not an evaluative study, identified a range of health and social benefits that can result from involving lay people in programme delivery. Box 4.1 categorises these benefits into three levels of outcomes.

Box 4.1: Three levels of outcomes for citizen involvement

Outcomes at an individual level

Changes can be understood in terms of improvements in the health of individual participants, both those delivering services as lay health workers and those receiving them. Outcomes can be educational (increases in knowledge, awareness or skills), behavioural (adoption of healthy lifestyles), social (improvements in social relationships) and empowerment (increases in individual confidence and capacity to act to improve health). They can reflect changes in physical or mental health status or even changes in the determinants of health, such as education or employability.

Outcomes at an organisational level

Lay involvement can lead to organisational outcomes, with public services better able to engage with the communities they wish to work with. Outcomes can include improved public health intelligence, enhanced skills of the professional workforce, improved relationships with service users, better organisational policy and redesigned services. These intermediate outcomes can lead in turn to better access to health and health care (eg increased uptake of screening services) and more appropriate use of health services, with potential for reduction of service costs.

Outcomes at a community level

Involving individuals in public health activity is a way of building community capacity and can lead to changes in communities. Rogers and Robinson (2004) argue that community engagement works through socialisation (internalising cooperative sociable standards), guardianship (looking after members of the community) and information flows between communities and public bodies. These processes can result in positive outcomes in relation to social capital (both

---

strengthening bonds within communities and strengthening internal and external networks), increased community capacity and resilience, changes to social or physical environments, and increased civic engagement.

A recent thematic evaluation of the community health champions programme (White et al, 2010b) found that outcomes for participants were often linked and tended to be framed in terms of social connectedness. For example, peer support from a community health champion might lead to increased confidence, which would enable someone to take part in regular exercise in a group, through which they would make friends and thereby reduce their social isolation, resulting in improved mental health. Neuberger (2008, p 14) argues that volunteering can become 'a virtuous circle, leading to more cohesive communities, higher levels of well being, and better use of people's potential'. Chapter Five provides examples of where engagement in a lay health worker role was a transformative experience and offered a gateway to opportunities for wider participation, new life skills, further education and employment. One expert witness talked about a developmental model:

> "I think breastfeeding is a really good example of where the developmental model can really take off because you have mums, through Children's Centres, who go to breastfeeding peer support groups, they breastfeed their children when maybe they wouldn't do, and then they get interested and become trained as peer supporters themselves, and do peer support training themselves. We have evidence … of mums then going on to train as midwives through further education and that's a developmental process. So actually you start off with somebody who maybe is not going to breastfeed who breastfeeds and ends up as a midwife." (Expert hearing 3)

What is the evidence base?

There are undoubted challenges in building an evidence base for community engagement (for further discussion, see Chapter Eleven) as it is regarded as a ubiquitous concept that few disagree with in principle, but, at the same time, its intangible results appear difficult to capture (Burton, 2009). A recent rapid evidence review examined the current evidence on the community health champion role, using a hierarchy of evidence that drew on systematic reviews, reviews of published evidence and expert reviews of similar roles such as lay health advisors (South et al, 2010c). Key findings included:

- **Evidence of increased knowledge and awareness of health issues.** For example, peer approaches for HIV prevention have been found to be effective at increasing HIV knowledge in developing countries (Medley et al, 2009).

- **Evidence on health behaviour change.** For example, a systematic review of peer nutrition education on dietary behaviours and health outcomes among the US Latino population found that interventions involving peer nutrition workers resulted in positive outcomes, including improved dietary intake with significantly lower intakes of saturated fat and increased consumption of fruits and vegetables, better food safety knowledge and skills, and increased levels of physical activity (Perez–Escamilla et al, 2008).
- **Evidence on increased individual capacity.** For example, Visram and Drinkwater (2005) reported positive outcomes in terms of confidence, self-esteem and empowerment, as well as other changes in personal health-related behaviour in their review of research and UK practice on lay health advisors, peer educators and health advocates.
- **Evidence of improved access to and increased uptake of services.** For example, a series of Cochrane Reviews of lay health workers in primary and community care report that lay health workers were effective at increasing uptake of immunisation in both adults and children, although the evidence was more mixed on lay involvement in screening (Lewin et al, 2005, 2006, 2010).
- **Evidence of improved health status.** For example, a US systematic review of community health workers involved in education and care of people with hypertension found positive outcomes associated with support from community health workers, including improvements in blood pressure control and health care use, such as appointment-keeping (Brownstein et al, 2007).
- **Evidence of impact on health care services.** For example, a systematic review of community health workers and care of people with diabetes reported on two studies where there was a decrease in emergency attendances in the treatment groups and one where there was a significant decrease in hospital admissions related to diabetes (Norris et al, 2006).
- **Evidence on benefits for volunteers.** For example, a systematic review carried out for Volunteering England found that the act of volunteering can have a range of positive outcomes in terms of improvements in self-rated health status, quality of life, ability to carry out activities of daily living, family functioning and social support, psychological distress, and depression (Casiday et al, 2008).

Overall, there is a good body of evidence demonstrating the effectiveness of lay health workers in promoting health and improving access to services. Much of the evidence originates from US interventions working with socially excluded or disadvantaged communities, which suggests that such approaches can be an effective tool in addressing health inequalities (see Chapter Eleven).

Value for money – what are the economic arguments?

As discussed earlier, one motivation for involving members of the public in delivering public health programmes can be to increase service capacity and promote more efficient use of scarce resources. These arguments have salience in a period of economic restraint and retrenchment of public services (see Chapter Two). Common-sense reasoning suggests that volunteer roles might offer a 'cheaper option' than delivery through a professional workforce. It is preferable to consider these issues in terms of value for money rather than cost savings as there are costs attached with supporting volunteers and paid lay workers. These costs include professional support to establish a project, recruitment, training, expenses, incentives and provision of ongoing support (Elford et al, 2002; Gaskin, 2003; Abbatt, 2005). Swider (2002, p 19) highlights the 'labor intensiveness' of community health worker programmes. These costs may be significant; Elford et al (2002, p 357) estimated that in a Popular Opinion Leader HIV intervention, training and support from the health promotion team added up to an average of 16.4 hours per week of professional time over 18 months.

While costs need to be taken into account, involving members of the public in delivery can still present an efficient use of health resources. Corluka et al (2009) found some evidence that lay health workers were more cost-effective in immunisation than comparative forms of delivery, although only three studies were included in the systematic review. Cost-effectiveness vignettes were prepared as part of the NICE review on community engagement (NICE Secretariat, 2007). One study showed that volunteer peer educators were more effective and less costly than experienced paid leaders in a group course promoting safe sex, but the authors pointed out that cost-effectiveness would diminish if changes in behaviour were not sustained over time.

Weighing up the true costs and benefits of citizen involvement in public health programme delivery is hampered because of a lack of evidence and the inherent difficulty in measuring value in these contexts. Brownstein et al (2007, p 445) pose the question: 'how does one place a monetary value on the characteristics and actions of laypeople [sic] from the community who, in many cases, volunteer to help others?'. The New Economics Foundation (NEF) public benefit model also offers a robust critique of traditional ways of looking at value for money (Ryan-Collins et al, 2007, p 13): 'Whether they are direct beneficiaries, their families or the wider community, the current VFM [value for money] model is blind to the resources that people and communities can add to making services not just cheaper, but better.'

New models are emerging that provide frameworks to assess those wider social and economic benefits and value for money. NEF has championed the Social Return on Investment (SROI) methodology (Nicholls et al, 2009). This is starting to provide evidence on the value of investing in community development, described by Alison Seabrooke as 'an early intervention which reduces the burden on the public purse' (NEF Consulting, 2010, p 1).

Moral and ethical arguments

So far, this chapter has set out the main rationales for involving lay people in programme delivery and demonstrated the existence of an evidence base to support social action. These arguments cannot be considered as ideologically neutral and it is vital that the moral dimensions are included in any assessment of the value of citizen involvement. Contrasting ideological perspectives are explored in more depth in Chapter Eleven and assumptions that voluntarism is necessarily associated with a neoliberal stance are challenged. This section provides a brief summary of some of the main rights–based arguments that support citizen involvement in health.

The right of people to participate in health was enshrined in the Alma-Ata declaration in 1978 (World Health Organization, 1978) and this provided an initial stimulus for the development of community health worker programmes (see Chapter Three). The World Health Organization defines health promotion as 'the process of enabling people to increase control over and to improve their health' (World Health Organization, 2009, p 1) and continues to advocate for community participation as a central strategy for health promotion. Participation is conceptualised not just as a process to support better health and health services, but also as a democratic right, a fundamental part of citizenship and a way to achieve empowerment (World Health Organization, 2002). Empowerment is a central construct as it concerns individuals and communities reversing factors that cause powerlessness and enhancing socially protective factors, such as social cohesion and community capacity (Wallerstein, 2002).

There are normative arguments about the value of volunteering to society, based on the dual notions of philanthropy (helping others) and reciprocity (giving mutual aid). Volunteering can be seen as an act of citizenship (Dingle and Heath, 2001) and therefore goes beyond helping governments meet their objectives to encompass advocacy and building the fabric of civil society (Dingle and Heath, 2001; Ware and Todd, 2002). Engagement can lead to articulation of social goals, the reversal of marginalisation and a challenge to professional power (Jauffret-Roustide, 2009). Expectations about active citizens are key to debates on the Big Society (Cabinet Office, 2011) and while communities are exhorted to 'play their part' in the context of a shrinking state, questions remain about the balance of responsibilities between the state and its citizens (see Chapter Two).

A further theme concerns the moral imperative to act to address health inequalities. The Marmot Review provided an assessment of the extent of health inequalities in England and a call for action (The Marmot Review, 2010a). In his introduction, Marmot makes no apologies for his stance advocating greater equity and social justice and calls it 'ideology with evidence' (The Marmot Review, 2010a, p 1). In The Marmot Review (2010a), community participation is presented as a strategy to develop healthy communities, where people have greater control over their own lives. Reduction of social isolation and building social capital in communities are identified as priority actions. Wallerstein (2002) contends that empowerment approaches are a legitimate strategy for reducing health inequalities because they build community capacity to improve equity and quality of life. It is argued elsewhere that the bridging role of volunteers, helping people achieve access to the health services and resources that they need and are entitled to, can be seen as an aspect of social citizenship (South et al, 2011a). Here, participation is a response to deficits in welfare provision, and there are questions about the fairness of expecting involvement from communities who bear the brunt of structural inequalities, which are explored further in Chapter Eleven.

Key points

- There are a number of justifications for citizen involvement in public health, based on the bridging role of lay health workers as a strategy to address health inequities, theoretical understanding of the value of peer-to-peer interventions, improved communication, increased service capacity and opportunities for service planning to be informed by better community intelligence.
- Engaging members of the public in delivering public health is linked to strategies for achieving social justice.
- Health benefits that result can be at the individual level, at the organisational level through developing services more attuned to community needs, and at the community level, with potential for stronger, more resilient, better-networked communities.
- There is a growing evidence base on lay health worker interventions and peer-based approaches, but more needs to be known about the balance between the investment needed to support people in their role and the social return on that investment.

FIVE

The lay perspective

Introduction

This chapter explores the perspectives of lay health workers and service users regarding members of the public taking on health improvement roles. There is a paucity of literature elucidating lay perspectives (Farquhar et al, 2008), particularly reporting the experiences of programme recipients. One of the primary aims of the People in Public Health study was to investigate consumer perspectives on these roles, thereby building knowledge in this area, and this chapter presents findings from interviews, expert hearings and workshops conducted as part of the study (South et al, 2009, 2010b). The chapter also draws on material from recent evaluative studies conducted by the authors, including a thematic evaluation of the role and activities of community health champions in the Altogether Better programme (White et al, 2010b) and evaluations conducted into the work of health trainers and health trainer champions (see Chapter Three; see also White et al, 2010a, 2011; White and Kinsella, 2011).

A systematic review, commissioned by Volunteering England, on the impact of volunteering on health (Casiday et al, 2008) concluded that volunteering can impact positively on many aspects of the volunteer's own health, including longevity, adoption of healthy lifestyles, ability to cope with their own ill health, family relationships, quality of life, social support and interaction, self-esteem, and sense of purpose. The review also demonstrated that volunteering can reduce stress and depression. The findings presented here support the conclusions of this review. This chapter discusses what motivates people to volunteer, what qualities and skills they need, what their volunteering may lead on to, and what barriers can prevent people from getting involved or progressing in volunteer roles. The chapter also explores the perspectives of service users on the experience of being supported by a volunteer rather than, or in addition to, a paid worker. The material is gathered from interviews, focus groups and workshops undertaken in the various studies, where the authors were privileged to listen to people who were, and are, making huge contributions to their communities. Their passion, commitment and level of engagement were inspiring and, where possible, their own words and stories have been used to bring the text alive.[1]

Motivations for volunteering

For some people, volunteering is only a small part of their lives, but for a sizeable number, it is a major and important part of their weekly, even daily, routine. The

People in Public Health study explored what motivates people to get involved and the case studies of public health projects provided an opportunity to look at motivation in some depth. As might be expected, motivations were varied, but there was consistency across the projects, with five key motivations emerging:

• Altruism – the desire to benefit others.
• Career pathway – volunteering as a stepping stone into work.
• Stage of life – being at a point where the 'time was right' to volunteer.
• Health and social benefits for the volunteer themselves.
• Having been a service user – motivated by either positive or negative experiences.

Not surprisingly, many people had a mixture of motivations, and what motivated them initially could be somewhat different from what gave them ongoing motivation to stay involved; nevertheless, altruism emerged as the strongest motivating factor, a finding supported by other research on volunteering (Brooks, 2002; Low et al, 2008). Public health roles were seen as appealing because of the opportunity to make a contribution to society. This theme was also reflected in the evaluation of community health champions (White et al, 2010b), where one participant clearly articulated how this was part of her philosophy of life:

> "[Becoming a community health champion] has certainly enhanced my quality of life especially when I see how much others can give to us and we have to give to others as well in turn. We all need each other in this life really and we don't gain anything by living in isolation."

While lay people volunteered without any expectation of gaining materially, for many, their public health role did lead to personal benefits, such as engagement in social activities or increased confidence. The following quotation illustrates that the desire to give back can bring much personal satisfaction:

> "I think it's a good opportunity for everybody really, gets them out of home and doing something of value. I had two strokes and I was stuck in doors lacking confidence … but meeting [the project worker] she got me out of it. I went on the health walks and I'm actually running the Tai Chi now which I'm so pleased about and it's got me out of the house and I'm out of the house more now and my husband doesn't see me very much because I'm so committed to my volunteer work."

Service users interviewed in the People in Public Health study appreciated that lay workers gave their time voluntarily because they wanted to be involved, and, for some participants, this distinguished them from paid workers:

"Well they want to be here for a start, professional people might only come for the money ... I think that's the main thing because they want to be here rather than get a wage cheque at the end of the week."

For some lay health workers, their primary motivation for volunteering was to help them in their career pathway. Taking on a public health role often helped to build confidence and skills, and opened up opportunities for training and personal development. For some, being active as a volunteer enabled them to gain the confidence to start looking for work:

"Honestly, if I'd seen the advert in the paper and I hadn't been volunteering and I hadn't got involved with health promotion, there's no way I would have applied for the job, it wouldn't even have entered my head."

In the community health champion evaluation for Altogether Better, there were some projects that focused on offering volunteering as part of a pathway into work, with considerable success. There is a tension, however, in recognising that volunteering can be a stepping stone to new opportunities and seeing its value solely as a means to enter the job market or to improve career prospects. At the People in Public Health expert hearings a member of the audience commented that Labour government policy was encouraging job centres to look differently on volunteering:

"That certainly came up in the ... event, the limitations of being unemployed or on some kind of benefit and being able to volunteer. And in a way that could be a good thing because it's about opening up employment opportunities for people who have put in a lot of voluntary work and developed a lot of skills and expertise and could do a really good job in a paid capacity. And in terms of their family income or lifestyle, that might be something that they really want. There's also then a danger of seeing volunteering as simply a route to employment rather than a good thing in its own right."

While individuals being able to progress from volunteer to paid roles is an undoubtedly positive outcome, this quotation highlights a potential area of concern that people may volunteer not so much for altruistic reasons, but to further their careers, or even because they are required to do so. The experience in Sheffield, where volunteering as community health champions is helping many back into employment, suggests that this is not the case. Volunteers are motivated by wanting to work with people, but need paid work because of their personal circumstances, and their experience as a community health champion helps them apply for jobs. Similarly, in the community health educators project described in

Chapter Eight, sessional payment helped people on low incomes to participate, but their primary motivation remained altruistic.

For those who were retired or unable to take up full-time employment because of family commitments or their own ill health, getting back to work clearly was not a motivation. It was more that the 'time was right', that is, they found themselves with time on their hands and a desire to give something back. One individual described moving to a village and becoming a volunteer walk leader because "I hadn't fully retired, I'd semi-retired and I wanted to do something, an activity like get into walking, something to keep you fit". Students were another group who potentially had free time to offer; one volunteer explained: "Well I'm a student and I have quite a bit of free time and I figured it would be better to do something useful than just sit at home and watch TV and I quite like doing volunteer work".

Public health roles were seen as providing health benefits. Many lay health workers had their own health concerns, including some with long-term conditions that meant they were unable to work. Becoming a lay health worker could aid recovery, give a sense of purpose and help individuals achieve a healthier lifestyle. Other individuals had originally joined projects with the hope that participation would improve or maintain their health and had ended up volunteering:

> "Well normally I used to go for walks, as I say I am a very active person, you know bringing up five children that helped, and I wanted to keep up with my health and I started with going for walks and from there I wanted to do a walk leading, voluntary walk leading, and I trained to be a walk leader."

The social aspects of volunteering could be a motivation. Some had previously experienced loneliness or social isolation and found that they made friendships through their roles. Others, such as students and the retired, welcomed the opportunities to meet new people. A sense of enjoyment and achievement was a motivating factor. One volunteer explained: "If you can make one person smile in a day it's worth everything ... and we have had a lot of people smiling".

Some volunteers were motivated by having been a service user and, having benefited from the service, then wanted to help others in a similar position. Others were motivated by a negative experience, or having witnessed people getting inadequate support. One breastfeeding peer support volunteer explained:

> "And it's something, breastfeeding, that I do feel quite passionate about and I do feel it's a real shame when you do speak to mums and, you know, I've got very good friends who, you know, gave up. Gave up's a bit of a harsh word but, you know, didn't manage to breastfeed as long as they wanted to because they didn't feel they got the support."

A member of the audience at one of the expert hearings observed that a desire to change things was a powerful motivation: "a lot of people get involved in something because something's gone wrong or something's not right or they're angry".

Arguably, it is what people do, what they contribute, that matters rather than their motivation, but it is important to understand what might encourage people to get involved, in order to build on that and thereby recruit and retain more volunteers.

Qualities and skills

This section looks at the views of service users and what they saw as the essential qualities of a lay health worker. It discusses the significance of social and communication skills, which were identified not just by service users, but by lay health workers and project staff, as essential to being an effective volunteer in a public health role. Building on this, the section explores whether service users and volunteers thought it important for lay workers to be 'peers' and what they meant by this. Service users were interviewed from three of the People in Public Health case study projects (Walking for Health, Neighbourhood Health and Breastfeeding Peer Support) (for more details, see the Appendix; for a more detailed discussion of results, see South et al, 2012). Examples from research with community health champions and health trainers are included where they complement the People in Public Health study.

In general, service users commented very positively on the qualities and skills that lay health workers brought to their roles. They talked about having high levels of trust in, and respect for, the lay health workers. People spoke of feeling cared for and supported and were appreciative of the generosity showed. For example, at a focus group in the Breastfeeding Peer Support project with women mainly of South Asian origin, some individuals viewed the peer supporter as a 'mother figure' and felt that they received personal support combined with culturally appropriate advice.

A range of important volunteer attributes, such as knowledge, skills and past experience, were identified through the People in Public Health study. One common theme was the importance of lay health workers having good 'people' skills, with service users valuing attributes like being approachable, non-judgemental, being a good listener and having patience:

> "They are the glue, aren't they, they keep us all together. [Name] is a great communicator, even though I haven't been for a few weeks, he gave me a call to see how I am, he makes you feel as though you are part of the group."

> "Well, they are really friendly and they are confident with us and we can talk to them and joke with them and everything, so it's like that.

> You can't be with outside people like that, they are like, well we know
> them so we can actually ask them and talk to them."

The absence of professional qualifications was not an issue for service users, as lay health workers were seen as offering something distinctive from health professionals. There were, however, different views on the extent and type of knowledge required in the roles. For example, in Walking for Health groups, some service users talked about the importance of local (geographical and historical) knowledge, while others identified the need for some basic level of health knowledge to cope with possible incidents. Similarly, in the Breastfeeding Peer Support project, one service user believed that individuals should have previous experience of breastfeeding if they were to become peer supporters, but in the focus group, the women emphasised the need for the peer support worker to be friendly, knowledgeable and able to interpret community languages. Language and cultural skills were considered necessary in order to access health information:

> "First of all she's bilingual and I know it's a breastfeeding group but
> we pick up so many different things as well whilst we're here. So just
> like health and different contraception and breastfeeding and you pick
> up on other things like cooking."

Being a peer

Differences in opinion about what constitutes a peer have been touched upon in Chapter Four. The World Health Organization (2007, p 1) recommends that lay health workers 'should be members of the communities where they work'. In the People in Public Health study, there were diverse views advanced about the need for the lay health worker to be drawn from within the community of interest, ranging from those who saw it as helpful but not at all necessary, through to those who perceived that shared identity was a critical factor. This debate is reflected in the literature reviewed for the study, where there has been some confusion about the term 'peer' and how it is used (South et al, 2010b). Peer status may be based on one or more matched characteristics, ranging from generic population categories such as age, through to more sophisticated concepts, such as experience of successful breastfeeding. Community health champions had similar debates in the workshops that were organised as part of the evaluation of the champion role in the Altogether Better programme (White et al, 2010b). Some champions were adamant that volunteers should come from the locality they worked in:

> "I think that's really important. I think the fact that there are very few
> health professionals, educational professionals who actually live in the
> area that they work in. That applies to a lot of inner city areas and
> they tend to live outside and come in. I think that creates a barrier to
> a certain degree, whereas people who live within that community, the

people you may see down at the shop or whatever and it's possibly easier to engage people in conversation and to build up trust. Whereas my experience of professionals isn't always like that at all, there's that distance, that geographical difference and maybe difference in terms of social class. So I think that makes a big difference to the way that champions are perceived."

Other champions emphasised shared experience with community members, which enabled them to build trust and rapport:

"Well I've lost two stone, which for me to be able to tell people who come, most of them know me from when I was bigger anyway, but they can see that I'm practically doing it and not just sitting there saying you need to lose weight and sat there being big. They know I've lost the weight so they know that I am doing my own steps and I'm doing it with them, so I can give them practical advice that I know does work."

Despite some difference of opinion, it was generally agreed that to be effective, champions needed to have sufficient in common with the communities they were working with in order to empathise with the people they were approaching, as well as being able to build trust. The health champion role was often about connecting with marginalised communities that professionals found 'hard to reach'. Being able to communicate effectively with people who might be nervous or mistrustful of professionals was identified as key and linked to being a peer:

"I think the biggest one [quality] is just being able to get on with people, it's just that communication in a way that engages people without being patronising or preaching. You know, they're just seen as one of the community, one of them, so, you know, can get close to people in a way that many professionals will never be able to do."

In summary, the skills and qualities brought to, and developed within, lay health worker roles are around life experience, combined with social, communication and language skills. These are complementary to professional skills and enable lay health workers to perform a bridging role. There is an evident gap between lay perspectives on valued skills and attributes and the competencies of levels 1 and 2 of the Public Health Skills and Career Framework (Public Health Resource Unit and Skills for Health, 2008) where lay health workers are placed, which suggests that only limited/low-level skills are needed. The People in Public Health study concluded that competency frameworks need to reflect the value of social skills and life experience in these roles, without edging towards inappropriate professionalisation. The arguments around how and why public health should be building on the assets within communities are discussed further in Chapter Twelve.

The volunteer journey

The Commission on the Future of Volunteering (2008, p 6) 'Manifesto for Change' describes volunteering as existing in 'a spectrum of involvement', with varying intensity of involvement from regular to episodic. The report uses the concept of a volunteer journey to describe both how people move into and out of volunteering across a lifespan and how their involvement can deepen and develop. The volunteer journey can also lead to people getting back into work and education. Paradoxically, while the benefits system still puts barriers in the way of volunteering, the government is increasingly encouraging people to take up a volunteer role to improve their own life chances as well as contribute to the Big Society (Cabinet Office, 2011; see also Chapter Two). This section looks at how volunteering can be a stepping stone to employment or training for some, but how others face barriers in just making the step into volunteering.

As discussed earlier, some people are motivated to volunteer in a public health role at least in part in the hope that this will improve their prospects of getting a job. Volunteering can give people a structure to their week, build skills and confidence, and, importantly, provide them with a reference. The People in Public Health study found that training courses could provide networking opportunities through which people could learn about job opportunities and start to gain confidence. As well as developing new skills, participation could also validate prior knowledge and experiences:

> "It's built up my confidence as well … it builds up your confidence and you're able to go and work, go off and do other things and it helps people come off the benefits and go into jobs and things."

The volunteer journey was about individual histories. Although volunteering was undoubtedly a stepping stone into employment for some, there were many other volunteers who never considered or wanted to go on to make a career based on their voluntary work. For some individuals, volunteering was a transformative experience. For those whose experiences had led to a downward spiral resulting in imprisonment or addiction to drugs or alcohol, volunteering could be part of the slow process of getting their lives back together, as illustrated by Box 5.1.

Box 5.1: A Sheffield Well-being story

Adrian could not wait to leave school, and joined the army at 16. A few years later, he was driving a tank and on operations in Bosnia. When Adrian left the army, he found life a struggle. He tried labouring and factory work, but went into a downward spiral, including problems with alcohol. Three years ago, Adrian came to Sheffield and began to turn his life around with the support of Healthy Cross Community Project in Southey. "I was keen to get fit again by going to the gym", he says, "and I started to volunteer at Healthy Cross. Then I became a

Health Champion." Adrian began by helping with the 'shopping squad', which takes isolated people shopping and helps them choose affordable, preferably healthy, food. He also helped out at festivals and community events, giving out information leaflets and making fruit kebabs and smoothies.

Before long, Adrian was helping to run the 'strollers' group that went walking in the Peak District, and taking a group rock climbing at the Works. He carried out risk assessments before the activities, and his ability and commitment led to staff giving him increasing amounts of trust and responsibility. When he heard that a swimming group needed a qualified lifeguard, he volunteered to 'train up'; he also got his minibus driver's certificate so that he could take groups out. Soon, he was also running a gym group and providing one-to-one support to a client wanting to improve his health and fitness. Adrian says: "I'm much fitter than I used to be, have learned to cook really healthy meals, don't drink or smoke. I have a real sense of well-being. I've turned my life around and know where I'm going." Adrian has just got a job as a support worker with Phoenix Futures in Barnsley – because of his work as a health champion. He says: "I have my dream job".

Source: Sheffield Well-being Consortium (no date[b]).

While volunteering is not transformational for everyone, it becomes an important part of people's lives, which benefits their health and well-being as well as providing a service to others. The reciprocal nature of volunteering (Baines and Hardill, 2008; Casiday et al, 2008) was reflected in the People in Public Health study's findings, where those who took on a lay health worker role often gained confidence, which contributed to subsequent life decisions and opened up new opportunities. Additionally, it was apparent that many service users were not always passive recipients, but often took more active roles in the project, such as helping out in the organisation and delivery of group activities or supporting other group members, or, indeed, volunteering in other areas of community life (South et al, 2012). For example, the trained volunteer would lead a walk, but a regular walker might volunteer to be the 'back marker'. This again fits with the concept of a spectrum of involvement. Enabling people to move from informal to formal roles and increasing the intensity of involvement may offer a key to sustainability (South et al, 2012).

Barriers to volunteering

Volunteers often start out as service users, but there are barriers to volunteering that deter people from making a contribution (Neuberger, 2008). Some of the service users interviewed spoke of personal circumstances preventing them from taking up a volunteer role. These included physical disabilities or health concerns, and the pressures of family commitments:

"Well that's the only thing, a lot of people have got commitments and they can't be bothered to do voluntary work 'cause they've got families, they've got children, grandchildren, they're running shopping and they're doing work for other people."

Red tape, such as Criminal Records Bureau (CRB) checks, and being asked to be on a committee were also seen as barriers. Formal processes of training and registration were major obstacles where there were literacy or language barriers:

"So to be a walk leader you need to write names and to take names and things like that. We both have difficulty with writing so it would be hard for us, so I don't think we'd be able to."

These comments by service users reflect the findings in other reviews of volunteering (Niyazi and National Centre of Volunteering, 1996; Gaskin, 2003). These barriers can effectively exclude some groups from volunteering at all (The Commission on the Future of Volunteering, 2008). Worries about impacts on benefits or being left out of pocket will also impact most on disadvantaged groups. At the third expert hearing, which focused on barriers, there was a call for clarity regarding conflicts between benefits and payments/incentives for lay people. A volunteer explained:

"In the voluntary sector, normally it's mostly people who are unemployed or in between jobs or things like that and they have to have social security or benefits and when you have a form to fill, you have to declare anything and then that comes off your benefits so that has actually made it a little bit difficult for people in the voluntary sector to actually come forward and those are the people who are wanting to do the voluntary work, so just thinking what could be helped in that situation because you have to declare everything on the form, even expenses." (Expert hearing 3)

In addition to these very practical barriers, the way public services operated could constrain the volunteer journey. A lay health worker giving evidence suggested that health professionals are the greatest barrier to lay involvement, as they perceive service change to be 'threatening'. She explained that:

"it's almost like saying they're not doing their job properly and we're not saying that. What we're saying is we're offering an enhanced service, we're here to work with you, but 95 percent of people don't like change. They're quite comfortable in their own comfort zone and if you suggest that they change their practice, they don't like it and the barriers go up."

Why professionals can feel threatened by volunteers is discussed in Chapter Eleven. A further barrier cited was the frequent absence of infrastructures to support lay people. In the expert hearings, Primary Care Trusts were criticised for having cumbersome bureaucratic processes that were difficult for lay people to navigate. A volunteer explained about the difficulties faced by her community group:

> "As a small group, we've got more hoops to jump through than any organisation. We have to account for every last penny, a big organisation doesn't have that same, 30 pounds for a report, you've got to practically price your staples up and that sort of stuff, that's how hard it is for people on the ground."

Some lay people experienced difficulties in their roles, which could prove barriers to retention. For example, where they were members of the community in which they worked, difficulties with gaining acceptance could impact on them individually:

> "And it can be anything down to the neighbours mocking you, look at that, 'she's a do-gooder getting out there and walking all the time' and you can become isolated, there are all sorts of factors."

Alongside the difficulties that lay people could experience, there could also be benefits when their association with a project was recognised. One volunteer explained: "If you name-drop ... 'I volunteer for [organisation]' ... I've generally found you get a bit of kudos, a bit of respect, a bit of 'Oh really?'".

This section has discussed, from a lay perspective, some of the reasons why people who want to gravitate to volunteering might feel unable to do so. Clearly, these are many and varied, some are to do with individual circumstances that prohibit people committing to a volunteer role, others are more to do with organisational procedures that get in the way. The case study projects described in Chapters Six to Nine had all developed ways of proactively dealing with some of these barriers, thereby supporting people in their roles. Issues for the recruitment and management of lay health workers are also discussed in Chapter Ten.

Concluding remarks

The primary motivation for people getting involved in public health roles is to help others, and, for many, their involvement becomes an important part of their lives, sometimes in life-changing ways. Lay people bring not just their altruism to their volunteer roles, but many qualities and skills that, as Chapters Six to Nine explore, are making a difference not just to their health and well-being, but to that of their communities. Service users appreciate support from someone who is giving their time freely and there are many roles that are more appropriately undertaken by a lay person than by a professional. However, members of the public face a range of barriers to getting involved. Sometimes, this is to do with individual circumstances, but organisational culture, professional protectionism and onerous bureaucratic processes are often obstacles to lay engagement. More attention is needed to address these issues, particularly with groups who experience social exclusion, if the potential for people to engage in promoting health is to be realised (The Commission on the Future of Volunteering, 2008; Department of Health, 2011b). Most importantly, it is vital that the voices of lay people themselves are heard so that their motivations and needs can be understood and any barriers they face to becoming more fully engaged in promoting health can be addressed.

Key points

- Lay perspectives on volunteering and lay health worker roles offer unique insights into the benefits resulting from engagement and the potential constraints on the volunteer journey.
- There are a range of motivations for taking on a public health role, but a desire to help others and give back is the strongest influence.
- Individuals bring valuable experiences, skills and qualities to public health roles. Shared identity can be very important; however, it is the ability to make connections with communities that is a vital feature of the lay health worker role.
- Volunteering can be a springboard for personal development and offer pathways into employment, education and further opportunities for participation.
- Opening up routes into volunteering would require services to address practical and organisational barriers.

Note

[1] Quotations are drawn from the People in Public Health study unless otherwise indicated.

SIX

Walking for Health – a case study

Chapters Six to Nine present four case studies conducted as part of the People in Public Health study, which illustrate how roles, relationships and support processes work on the ground. The case studies were chosen to represent different approaches to involving lay people in the delivery of public health programmes and also diversity in terms of types of organisation and communities. More detail on the case study methods, sampling and analysis can be found in the Appendix. These case studies, as presented here, are not intended to provide comprehensive descriptions of the projects. Instead, the authors have chosen to present key issues emerging from the data in a thematic way to illuminate some of the most significant themes for public health practice. Real-life examples and verbatim quotations are used to illustrate some of the dilemmas and challenges faced by those engaged in public health activity, whether at a strategic, operational or community level; however, care has been taken to protect the anonymity of respondents by not using project names, locations, specific role titles or individual names.

Introduction

Walking for Health is a national initiative promoting community-based health walks, coordinated until recently through Natural England (Natural England, 2011b), and endorsed by the NHS (Department of Health, 2009). As a public health intervention, Walking for Health has achieved considerable success in terms of the scale of volunteer involvement to support wider participation in health (The Countryside Agency, 2005). The case study presented in this chapter focuses on the organisation and delivery of a local scheme operating across one Primary Care Trust, and the experience of being part of Walking for Health is explored through interviews with practitioners, volunteer walk leaders and participants. Walking schemes offer a simple model of community-based peer support, with volunteers acting independently following initial training. The chapter highlights choices over maintaining an infrastructure to support volunteers, and approaches to managing risk. The responsibilities of the walk leader role are examined and evidence is presented of deeper engagement processes at work in communities. The chapter starts with a summary of the main features of the Walking for Health initiative, prior to more detailed description of the local scheme that formed the case study.

Background

The Countryside Agency (now Natural England) together with the British Heart Foundation established the Walking Your Way to Health (now called Walking for Health) initiative in 2000 as a means of increasing physical activity in the sedentary population. At the time of the study, Walking for Health was coordinated by Natural England and was receiving some Department of Health funding to widen participation.[1] While some of the walks are led by health professionals and other practitioners, such as park wardens, it is volunteer walk leaders organising regular walks in their community who are the backbone of the initiative. Volunteers receive a standard one-day training session covering practical advice on how to lead a health walk, the benefits for health, route planning and risk assessments, completing the paperwork, and available resources (Walking for Health Team Natural England, 2011). Once trained, the volunteer walk leader role involves planning routes and supporting participants on the walk, ensuring everyone returns safely. There is usually another volunteer who acts as a 'back marker' by walking at the rear of the group. Although walk leaders may promote the benefits of walking, their role does not extend to providing health education, peer counselling or personalised support.

Since its inception, Walking for Health has grown rapidly and achieved a scale and reach not often seen in UK public health programmes. A review of local evaluations found that a wide range of health and social benefits were reported and the volunteer model was found to be sustainable with support (The Countryside Agency, 2005). In 2010, there were over 11,000 active walk leaders, many of whom are volunteers, and more than 63,000 people regularly taking part in health walks (Natural England, 2011b). Walking for Health attracts more women than men (72% to 28%, respectively) and three quarters are aged over 55 years (Natural England, 2011b).

Walking has been described as the 'easiest, most accessible, cost effective, and enjoyable way for most people to increase their physical activity' (Heron and Bradshaw, 2010, p 3). The establishment of lay-led walking groups therefore appears to offer a transferable model for encouraging wider engagement in health improvement. Attention has been on the effectiveness of volunteer-led walking schemes as a means of increasing physical activity with the sedentary population and there is a need for more evidence on impact (Lamb et al, 2002; National Institute for Health and Clinical Excellence, 2006; IPSOS Mori, 2011). Walking programmes can bring social benefits and these have been found to reinforce participation (South et al, 2011b). The Walk and Talk scheme for older people in Australia, for example, found that 55% of respondents were motivated to take part by the chance to meet people (Jones and Owen, 1998). Lay health workers can provide social support and supervision for participants of physical activity interventions (Westhoff and Hopman-Rock, 2002). Plescia et al (2006) identify the ability of the lay health advisors to form strong relationships with other stakeholders as a factor in a Lay Health Advisor programme in North Carolina, which included neighbourhood walking groups.

Walking for Health – a case study of a local scheme

Walking for Health was a natural choice for a case study because it offered a transferable model of involving volunteers. It represented an example of community-based peer support that was characterised by minimal professional involvement, in contrast to projects where lay health workers received more intensive training and supervision. The case study chosen was a district-wide Walking for Health scheme within one Primary Care Trust that was coordinated through the NHS, but with some local authority involvement. The overall scheme aimed to encourage people to take up walking, either as part of a group walk or independently. In line with the national initiative, there was a mix of delivery partners; some of the walks were led by health professionals or paid workers, but a major component was the training of volunteer walk leaders who then went on to lead community walks. Walk leaders received a short one-day training session giving practical advice on leading walks and running a group, basic first aid training, and information on how to do risk assessments. There were around 60 regular walks available across the district, based in both urban and rural areas, and varying in distance and group ability. Most walks were open to all, but there were some closed groups, for example, women-only walks. The original remit was increasing physical activity and general health improvement, but, recently, the emphasis within the Primary Care Trust had shifted to obesity and weight management.

The case study offered an opportunity to explore changing patterns of infrastructure support. In the early days of the Walking Your Way to Health initiative, the district, then served by four Primary Care Trusts, had received some funding from the Countryside Agency, via the Big Lottery, to pilot walking groups. Some of the first groups were set up in disadvantaged neighbourhoods, and some successfully engaged women of South Asian origin. Walk coordinator posts were later established by some of the Primary Care Trusts, supported by funding from the Countryside Agency. The coordinator role was to promote Walking for Health, recruit, train and support walk leaders, and organise local walks. Following organisational changes where the four Primary Care Trusts merged, a district-wide walk coordinator post was established, but, in 2008, funding for the post was withdrawn, leaving local walking groups without a central coordination and support facility. As part of the move away from service delivery to a commissioning role for Primary Care Trusts, Walking for Health was moved from public health to provider services and placed within the Obesity Prevention programme.

Interviews were conducted in 2009 with a range of stakeholders with either current or past experience of the scheme. The sample comprised 10 staff (practitioners with experience of coordinating or delivering the scheme), 10 volunteer walk leaders and three external partners, two from the local authority and one from Natural England. A number of practitioners had practical experience as walk leaders and some were able to give a historical perspective on the development of the local scheme. The research team was also given access to three established walking groups, one of which involved women from the South Asian community, and interviews or focus groups were conducted with 20 group members (referred to as service users). Findings from the case study include themes about the experience of walking groups and organisational themes around coordination, engagement and support, which are discussed first.

Outreach and engagement

Mirroring the growth of the national initiative, the local Walking for Health scheme had been successful in recruiting volunteers, with over 200 individuals undergoing walk leader training (although not all those completing training went on to lead a walk group), and had a track record of engaging diverse communities, including minority ethnic populations. Much of the recruitment was done through word of mouth, with walk coordinators and project workers doing outreach through various networks. Some publicity was distributed through community projects so that people looking for community courses or for voluntary experience could access information. Just seeing people walking in a group could be a stimulus and engagement was in essence an informal and pragmatic activity:

> "Obviously, some people just come along to do the walks and then go home, but there are others who are more involved and they maybe do a bit of promoting in the community and get people to come along. Not all, but some I ask, are interested in doing the basic walk leader's course and then being in a position to either assist or deliver walks themselves." (Staff)

The motivations of volunteers varied, some wanted to give something back to the community or simply enjoyed walking with other people to keep fit. Others, mainly younger age groups, could get valuable work experience. Reflecting some of the trends of volunteer engagement in health walks (The Countryside Agency, 2005), many of the walk leaders were reported to be retired and the time was therefore right for them to take on this role. Enjoyment and personal benefits did not necessarily conflict with more altruistic motivations (see Chapter Five), as one volunteer explained: "I enjoy walking so I want to introduce other people to enjoy walking".

There was no formal selection process, just a chat about the role with a walk coordinator. Criminal Record Bureau (CRB) checks were not required because "they're never on their own with an individual, they're always in a group, they're not going into people's houses" (external partner). In fact, many of those interviewed had undergone CRB checks because of other roles and did not see this as barrier.

While the overall picture was one of successful engagement, including with some groups deemed 'hard to reach', there were still barriers to volunteer involvement that were discussed by volunteers, practitioners and by walking group members. Literacy was identified as a significant barrier because of the training and registration processes. There were also language barriers where communities did not speak English as a first language and this was despite having access to practitioners who spoke other community languages and were able to translate as required in training:

> "Literacy. Well I think the things that put people off are the forms and stuff and it puts them off. Yes, because a lot of people have got the skills to do the activity but they might not have the literacy and they're not going to say 'I'm not doing it because I can't fill the form out because I can't spell and I can't write'. And there's languages as well. There's paperwork, registers for putting people's names down and it's surprising how many people can't do it particularly round here." (Staff)

One theme, also reflected in the other case studies, was the extent of commitment required to be a volunteer and whether this was compatible with family or work commitments. Given the short training and the standard delivery model, it might be assumed that the role was relatively undemanding, but this was not the case. Walk leaders were seen as carrying considerable responsibilities and the level of responsibility deterred some from taking up the role. Walking group participants did, however, take active roles within the group, such as distributing publicity or offering to be a back marker (South et al, 2012). One walking group member explained why they felt unable to be a walk leader:

> "Yes, I think it's health things really. I don't see very well, I wouldn't want to be in charge of a big group like today. I'd be worried about counting heads and things although I could very well do some of it. I'm fine to stay at the back and make sure there's nobody behind and that's fine." (Service user)

An infrastructure for supporting volunteers

The value of a supportive infrastructure to sustain volunteer involvement was highlighted throughout this case study. The volunteer leaders encouraged, organised and supported participation in the walking groups, often taking on extra responsibilities such as giving people lifts, and, in many ways, the activity within walking groups was self-sustaining. Nonetheless, there was a role for public health practitioners, and, more specifically, the walk coordinator, in supporting the activity on the ground, and this role included:

- collecting the walk registers;
- providing any leaflets or information that the walk leaders required;
- helping with administration, such as applying for small grants; and
- acting as a point of contact if problems arose.

This was often done very informally. One practitioner described phoning to check things were going well, or alternatively popping into the group: "it's just nice to keep in touch with them really but it doesn't happen really often".

The changes in scheme coordination, prompted mainly by wider organisational changes in the local health service, provided a point of comparison. One issue raised in the interviews was the value of networking meetings. When a walk coordinator had been in post, regular meetings were held in different localities where walk leaders could discuss walk routes and share general information. This was seen as a valuable support mechanism to keep people linked in and both practitioners and walk leaders were unhappy that the meetings had stopped.

Support was regarded as an essential factor in sustainability. Although the walk coordinator post was not about providing intensive support, a strong theme was the value of regular contact. The loss of the post was seen as having a negative impact on motivation and some walk leaders keenly felt the lack of support, with one, in fact, resigning. Some walk leaders also wanted better access to training or to practitioners who could help organise community health activities. While the Primary Care Trust still commissioned the scheme, the majority of the walk groups were left to be self-sustaining:

> "Well, the support weren't there. There was no support there. You just can't leave somebody high and dry. I mean if somebody have had rang up and said 'Look this is the situation, we've run out of money or we're not doing that anymore, we're going on to this', I'd probably have said 'Well I totally disagree with what you're doing' or whatever but there was none of that. And I'm thinking they just are not keeping in touch." (Volunteer)

A component of support for volunteering is the payment of expenses to recompense any expenditure occurred. Walking for Health is a volunteer scheme and volunteer walk leaders interviewed were happy to contribute because of the personal enjoyment of walking or giving back to the community. While it might be considered essential that these volunteer walk leaders were not out of pocket, which was something practitioners were keen to avoid, hidden expenses, such as the use of mobile phones or buying refreshments, could be difficult to claim back. In the past, a straight payment of £10 for each walk undertaken had been offered to cover expenses in some areas. This strategy was felt to encourage participation where people were unemployed and also provided an indication of the value of their contribution, but there was a risk of conflicts with welfare benefit claims. At the time of the interviews, this payment had been withdrawn but it did provoke discussion in terms of the difficulties that might be faced by those on low incomes. Various different stakeholders raised the question of fairness and the fact that a small payment indicated some value, particularly given the time commitments and the responsibilities of the walk leader: "I don't look for appreciation but it would be nice if we did get some [payment], that's like a slap in the face" (volunteer). Others recognised the distinctive nature of the voluntary contribution: "someone that is doing it for nothing who absolutely loves it will somehow bring another dimension to our walks" (service user). The findings illustrate how the issue of rewards is complex and relates to how people perceive the role and the extent of responsibilities (see Chapter Ten).

Independence and risk

Once trained, walk leaders acted independently in terms of the organisation of walks (see Table 6.1). The role included risk-assessing the routes, planning a timetable of walks and making decisions with regard to weather conditions and ensuring the safety of the walkers. The back marker role for slower walkers was also crucial for safety. Part of the initial training was on basic first aid[2] and all walk leaders carried a first aid kit. They also had responsibilities for getting walkers to complete a health questionnaire indicating existing health conditions and for keeping that information confidential. The issue of walk members with poor health was a concern for some, both professional and lay. Volunteer walk

Table 6.1: The walk leader role

Responsibilities of a walk leader	Knowledge, skills and attributes
Core roles:	**Local knowledge:**
– Lead walks in small groups	– Knowledge of good routes
– Organise walk programme	– Knowledge of local environment and history
– Plan new routes and do risk assessments	– Knowledge of local networks (which can help
– Take register and get new walkers to complete Outdoor Health Questionnaire	access hard-to-reach groups)
– Welcome new walkers	**Basic knowledge of health:**
– Carry a first aid kit	– First aid skills
– Ensure everyone returns safely	**Communication skills:**
	– Being a good listener
Additional roles:	
– Act as role models in community – encouraging people to walk	**Social skills:**
– Give out positive health messages about walking	– Being good with people
– Publicise walks	– Friendly and approachable
– Encourage people to gel in the walking group	– Displaying empathy and patience
– Highlight areas of local interest – historical or geographical features	**Language skills (where appropriate)**
	Non-professional status
	Commitment and enthusiasm:
	– Affinity for the place and people in an area
	Being trusted:
	– Able to respect confidentiality

leaders were insured through Natural England, but accidents were reported as a rare occurrence.

Although the short health walk was in nature a simple health intervention, the role of the walk leaders was seen as a very responsible position, and one that walking group members in particular saw as involving duties of caring. Walk leaders also had a role in bringing people together and encouraging participation. One walk leader described the role as "to encourage people to try and spend time with one another", while a walking group member stated: "they are the glue aren't they, they keep us all together". There was a tension between what was seen as a high level of responsibility for others and the health walk as a social event. A balance had to be struck based on common sense:

> "I mean you could go all the way to doing group assessments like they do in schools when they take groups of children out. That totally negates exactly where they are going to be, but they are actually in the role of the supportive friend in terms of doing this and would you expect a supportive friend to take you somewhere totally inappropriate? You'd expect them to use their common sense." (Staff)

Passion and commitment were part and parcel of being a volunteer walk leader, but there was a risk of volunteers being zealous about walking and they could on occasion "go outside their remit and become too involved, too intrusive" (staff). One example was given of a practitioner having to speak to a walk leader who had made a walker feel uncomfortable about their weight. Some of the practitioners interviewed highlighted the issue of reliability and the perception that the same degree of "control" could not be exercised over volunteers as within professional services. General practitioners (GPs) were reported to be "scared" of referring and worried about claims if people tripped over.[3] Ultimately, volunteer walk leaders were not expected to act as quasi-health professionals and the consensus was that risks were, in fact, small:

> "I guess there would inevitably be a potential concern about maintaining a consistent quality and standard of delivery, which you can partially overcome by training and development. But, even so, when you involve people that aren't part of an organisation, you are reliant upon them as individuals to stay on message and to have the right information and to portray a professional image of the organisation that they're representing, which is something that you can't control as much as if they're directly employed, of course. But it's a pretty small risk because the people that tend to volunteer tend to be committed and passionate about what they do anyway." (External partner)

An affinity with the community

The question of what lay health workers bring to public health is one that dominated the People in Public Health study. The mixed economy of provision, with both lay and professional walk leaders, allowed the research team to explore the value of the lay contribution. The concept of 'lay' also needed to be unpacked, as the extent to which walk leaders were peers and what that meant in the context of local communities was of interest.

The role of the volunteer walk leader was complex and carried significant responsibilities, covering aspects of organisation, safety, care and socialisation (see Table 6.1). Walk leaders needed to have a variety of skills and attributes, not only organisational skills and an interest in walking, but social and communication skills in order to facilitate participation and help the group gel:

> "They don't need to be looking at maps to navigate their way around, they are quite simple health walks, and I think, yeah, good social skills and being able to talk to people, and because you have to understand that maybe everyone is not as fit as them and just taking those things into account. So social, quite understanding and aware of what other people want and how to communicate, quite chatty and good at giving support and assistance." (Staff)

Commitment was important and walk leaders were often described as being passionate about walking and therefore acting as a role model in the community. Walking group members frequently described their walk leaders as approachable and caring, and with natural empathy for people.

The question of how much walk leaders needed to be identified with the local community was discussed. Being a peer could help those who were unsure of participation, for example, it was suggested that being of a similar age might help people feel comfortable to join in. The notion of shared identity and language also had some salience within the walking group with women of South Asian origin, but trust and social ties were most important here:

> "We're faces that they see every day so we have a relationship with every single lady so when we say to the ladies 'Will you come?', sometimes they don't want to come for a walk but we'll say to them 'Just come along and if you don't like it you don't have to do it' and they'll say 'OK then, we'll come' and then they'll come every week because they have a relationship with us and trust." (Volunteer)

Volunteer walk leaders often brought insight into the local community, knowledge of social networks and also geographical knowledge of the place. All of these attributes contributed positively to the experience of engagement in the health

—

walk and helped services access communities. This lay dimension not only increased service capacity, but also brought something distinctive:

> "'I think they have an affinity with the area, and often have a greater affinity with the people and an understanding of the needs of the people … I think they can often encourage people to participate that you wouldn't get if you were just using a professional network of officers." (External partner)

Acknowledgement of the value of the lay contribution did not imply that professional provision was inappropriate. Professional input gave Walking for Health credibility in some communities; therefore, a mix of provision was deemed important. In one of the walking groups where the walk leader was employed by the local authority, one walking group member argued that there were "pros and cons" to both ways because professionals were able to access agency resources, such as minibuses, but another spoke of the importance of being rooted in the locality, whether professional or lay.

The benefits of engagement

The Walking for Health initiative was designed as an intervention to increase levels of physical activity in the sedentary population. In the case study district, the local Primary Care Trust was the lead organisation and Walking for Health had been moved to sit within the obesity prevention team. The implications of this, combined with the shift in public health from provider to commissioning services within the Primary Care Trust, meant that the scheme was in the process of being commissioned as a weight management intervention with targets around the reduction of obesity. One practitioner explained the limitations of this approach as walks for mental health and social well-being were no longer seen as part of the remit.

In contrast to the target-driven world of the NHS, the majority of respondents described the wider benefits of health walks and frequently talked about the value of participation in terms of social outcomes rather than physical health. Both lay and professional stakeholders spoke of the personal benefits of becoming a walk leader, including:

- enjoyment;
- personal development;
- having a sense of achievement or purpose;
- meeting other people in the community;
- being part of a social group;
- being able to maintain personal fitness; and
- influencing family members to go walking.

Walk leaders often grew in confidence and the ability to speak to other people. Practitioners talked about the value of the experience in terms of employability and examples were given of people stepping into other community roles or on to a job. Sometimes, changes could be quite dramatic, for example, moving on from long-term mental illness to employment or learning communication skills to be able to represent community views. One practitioner who had previously been a volunteer walk leader explained the significance of taking on a volunteer role:

> "It's not just about the community, it's also about that lay person and again the skills that they could learn for career progression, whether back into education or back into work ... if they've never worked before. It gives them that confidence 'Well if I can do it as a volunteer, I can do it'." (Staff)

Evidence of walking groups as a mechanism for deeper engagement leading in turn to wider benefits was reflected across all the interviews. Volunteer walk leaders were a vital part of the delivery of physical activity sessions in the district, but their role was not purely functional. Walk leaders helped people participate in walks and overcome barriers that prevented them from walking, such as anxieties, fear of crime or lack of confidence. The social benefits of being in a group were motivating in terms of reinforcing regular participation: "you feel comfortable with the people you are walking with and also comfortable about the walking". Participants spoke of direct benefits relating to the reduction of social isolation, developing friendships, improved mental health and developing a feeling of belonging within a community. One walking group member explained the impact:

> "Well I moved to [name] nine years ago and I find it very hard to get to know people, how do you meet people, and I used to get very depressed actually. I never said 'Hello' to anyone, there was never a familiar face and I wanted to feel I belonged, and after joining the group I do feel like I belong. I feel I have an investment in the area whereas before I felt like I was just someone who'd moved here." (Service user)

Walk leaders helped raise awareness of the local area, pointing out new places or interesting historical buildings, and sometimes signposted people to other services or organised other health activities. Walking groups were seen to be a positive exercise choice for women from the South Asian community as groups provided safety and were seen as acceptable to older relatives. One practitioner who had successfully developed a number of walks for women of South Asian origin explained the wider impact in terms of changes in lifestyle that can result:

> "Wherever you go in the parks you'll see people walking and now some of them are doing fast walks and running and you see ladies with

traditional clothing with full head scarves but with bright white trainers on. It's so incongruous but the message is there and it's stuck." (Staff)

What does this model offer?

Walking for Health is an interesting example of volunteering in public health. It shows the potential to incorporate volunteer action into a simple delivery model and to scale that involvement up. This case study illuminates some of the facilitating factors that appear to support successful engagement. The volunteer walk leader role was the lynchpin of the programme. Without volunteers, delivery of the range of walks in the district would have been impractical. Furthermore, volunteer walk leaders were critical to the processes of engagement as they raised awareness of walking, encouraged people to join the groups, enhanced the experience and made people feel welcome and comfortable (South et al, 2012).

Walking for Health is a public health intervention that is focused on a single lifestyle issue. The delivery mode is uncomplicated; however, it should not be assumed that the volunteer walk leader role is undemanding. Instead, the case study shows that the role is complex, involving different processes of engagement to produce a functioning walking group where members support each other. A range of skills, both social and organisational, are required, as well as the capacity to undertake independent action. Responsibilities are not insignificant; nonetheless, there was a consensus that a common-sense approach to the management of risk could be achieved.

The benefits of a deeper engagement brought value to services, to community members and to the volunteers themselves. Social benefits from walking, such as reduction of social isolation, are health outcomes in themselves (Heron and Bradshaw, 2010) and may hold the key to engagement in physical activity (Jones and Owen, 1998). There was a mismatch between acknowledgement of the wider health and social benefits and the NHS framework of obesity targets. The conclusion here is that framing simple interventions in a narrow functional way misses the potential for public services to access communities and to build stronger communities through supporting voluntary action.

The case study illuminates a further issue around the need for organisational infrastructure to support volunteer activity. Where it worked well, support involved a short practical training session that was fit for purpose, informal community-based recruitment strategies, central coordination, access to some professional support and opportunities to network. These systems were not over-complicated or resource intensive, but helped keep volunteers engaged, motivated and supported. The withdrawal of that support through changes in the commissioning process was seen to impact negatively on volunteers. The issue of the payment of expenses was another complex issue with few easy answers, and this is discussed further in Chapter Ten. In summary, there is a need to actively address support needs and not to underestimate the lay role. One practitioner highlighted the potential to dismiss the programme as "it's easy, just walking" and concluded that "where we have gone wrong is we don't recognise the importance of a lay role and we don't actually give people the necessary support so that they can fulfil that role properly".

Key points

- The national Walking for Health initiative has been successful at recruiting large numbers of volunteers who lead health walks in their community. This case study of a local scheme explored the volunteer walk leader role and how this supported engagement in group walks.
- The walk leader role came with responsibilities in terms of independently organising the walks and supporting the participants, and many walk leaders demonstrated a high level of commitment to the role.
- The case study provides evidence of the importance of central coordination and light-touch volunteer support to enable people to feel supported in their roles.
- Participation, whether as a walk leader or group member, brought a range of social and health benefits, including reduction of social isolation, improved mental health and developing a feeling of belonging within a community.

Notes

[1] In April 2012, the national management of Walking for Health transferred to the Ramblers, working in partnership with Macmillan Cancer Support.

[2] The Walking for Health standard training package does not include first aid training but local coordinators often arrange additional first aid or 'Heartstart' training to be made available to volunteer walk leaders.

[3] Walking for Health is endorsed by the Medical Protection Society.

SEVEN

Sexual health outreach – a case study

There is a long tradition of using peer-based interventions in sexual health promotion, particularly in relation to HIV/AIDS prevention (Janz et al, 1996; Medley et al, 2009). This chapter presents findings from a case study of a sexual health outreach project that worked within the gay community to promote uptake of sexual health screening services. Volunteers were involved in supporting a community-based screening service for men who have sex with men and undertook peer education in gay bars and clubs. This small sexual health outreach project is of interest not only because it illustrates lay involvement within a community of identity rather than place, but also because it highlights some interesting issues about boundaries, roles and relationships within a community where health inequalities arise from stigmatisation and marginalisation of health needs (Daley, 2006). The chapter evidences some good practice in relation to support, training and development throughout the volunteer journey. The chapter starts by giving a brief overview of peer education approaches to promote sexual health within lesbian, gay, bisexual and transsexual (LGBT) communities.

Peer education in sexual health

Peer education methods and related approaches are used as the basis for sexual health promotion interventions, predominantly around prevention of sexually transmitted infections (STIs). It is argued that peers, sharing a common identity with the 'target community', will be able to communicate directly by using a common language and individuals will be more receptive to health messages from people who are perceived to share social norms, attitudes and experiences (Hart, 1998; Parkin and McKeganey, 2000). For public health, a further justification is the ability of peers to reach communities that are marginalised or underserved (McQuiston and Uribe, 2001). There is some evidence of effectiveness in relation to increased knowledge of HIV (Medley et al, 2009), condom use (Grinstead et al, 1999) and uptake of sexual health services (Williamson et al, 2001). Peer educators may be able to overcome barriers related to the sensitive or even taboo nature of some sexual behaviours, for example, distributing information in 'public sex environments' (French et al, 2000). However, in a peer-based intervention for male escorts, the issue of confidentiality was found to be a concern for men, some of whom suggested that due to embarrassment, 'outsiders' might, in fact, be a more appropriate source of information (Ziersch et al, 2000).

The National Institute for Health and Clinical Excellence (NICE) recommend that commercial venues where men who have sex with men meet should be used to promote HIV testing (National Institute for Health and Clinical Excellence,

2011). For sexual health initiatives within LGBT communities, there has been a tradition of outreach approaches located within social settings. For example, Stevens (1994) describes a peer education intervention run in bars and clubs where bisexual and lesbian women met. Her ethnographic study found that the peer educators were 'adeptly attuned' (Stevens, 1994, p 1575) to the knowledge and support needs of women and were accepted in those settings, and some women reported that the presence of peer educators served to reinforce messages. This notion that peer-based interventions have potential to influence cultural norms of behaviour is also the basis of the Popular Opinion Leader approach, which was trialled in the gay community in California. This model is predicated on the theory (based on Roger's Diffusion of Innovations theory) that positive behaviour change – here, around safer sexual practices – can be promoted and endorsed by opinion leaders, who are popular, well-known individuals with some social standing in a community (Kelly et al, 1992; Kelly, 2004). The Popular Opinion Leader model was not successfully transferred to a UK context when it was run in London gyms frequented by gay men, partially because of difficulties of recruitment and retention (Elford et al, 2002).

Sexual health outreach – a case study

The sexual health outreach project for men who have sex with men was selected as a peer education case study in the People in Public Health study because peer-based sexual health promotion featured strongly in the UK literature and because the project offered the opportunity to look at lay health worker roles within a community of identity that was not defined by social class. The sexual health outreach project was one of a number of activities run by a voluntary sector organisation working to address the sexual health of gay and bisexual men. The organisation's work was underpinned by a community development approach that sought to engage groups and individuals from various communities across the region, although much of the work was based in urban areas. Support and information was available for men who have sex with men through a wide variety of services, including support groups, youth projects, counselling services and telephone helplines. Like many voluntary sector organisations, activities were funded through a mix of public sector contracts, from both Primary Care Trusts and local authorities, and community donations.

The sexual health outreach project was part of a community-based sexual health service targeted at men who have sex with men and commissioned by the local Primary Care Trust. Rapid HIV testing, screening for chlamydia and gonorrhoea, and hepatitis A and B vaccinations were all provided in non-clinical settings. The project initially operated from the voluntary organisation's offices, but in order to improve access to the service, screening and immunisation (but not HIV testing) were taken out to bars and clubs on the 'gay scene' and, at the time of the research, the project was running one night a week in a number of commercial gay scene venues in the city centre, including licensed premises and events where LGBT communities socialised. In the early days, the services were delivered solely by staff employed by the organisation together with sessional nursing staff, but the following year, volunteers were introduced to increase service capacity as staff were reportedly struggling to cope with demand. In 2008, a volunteer coordinator was recruited to support volunteers, including in other volunteer roles within the organisation.

A small team of volunteers supported paid staff in outreach and related activities (see Box 7.1). The primary role of volunteers was to raise awareness of sexual health services and provide information on how to access them. There were protocols in place that delineated the volunteer role in outreach. Interviews were conducted with three volunteers and six staff (some of whom had previously been volunteers), including nurse practitioners, community development workers and the volunteer coordinator. Additional interviews were conducted with a strategic lead in the health service with responsibility for commissioning, and partner organisations who delivered linked screening services. It was not possible to interview bar owners and clients in the gay scene because of the sensitive nature of the outreach programme.

Box 7.1: Roles of volunteers and staff in the sexual health outreach project

Volunteer roles
- Promoting the screening service in commercial gay scene venues.
- Providing service users and potential service users with information about community testing.
- Recruiting individuals to the screening service and taking urine samples.
- Giving out information and answering questions about sexual health, including STI transmission, treatment and prevention.
- Helping with condom-packing and assisting with administration, such as filling in forms with service users.
- Serving drinks and talking to service users who were attending for HIV testing at the organisation's offices.
- Signposting individuals to other services within the organisation or to other services and groups.

Roles of professional staff
- Undertaking outreach alongside volunteers.
- Supporting the volunteers and providing professional advice.
- Giving hepatitis immunisations.
- Pre- and post-test HIV counselling.

Volunteer pathways

Perhaps more than in any of the other case studies, there was a sense of a process whereby becoming part of the organisation as a volunteer was only the start of a journey that involved personal development and sometimes progression to other roles, both paid and unpaid, within the organisation. The three volunteers who were interviewed were all in their early 20s. One had volunteered with the ultimate aim of obtaining a paid job within the organisation and this had given him a chance to explore how the organisation worked and get a "foot in the door". One was a student who felt he had some free time to volunteer, whereas the other volunteer described wanting to get involved because he was new to the area and regarded it as a good way to meet people. While individual motivations differed, it was evident that volunteering also involved making a positive choice, one that was based primarily on altruism. The notion of wanting to give back to the community could be seen by the fact that, according to one member of staff, roughly four in five of the staff and volunteers were also service users.

Volunteers and staff frequently spoke of a commitment to the community and also a sense of enjoyment:

> "I was looking for volunteer work in general and this was something that actually interests me and I wanted to do something useful for the community, even though it sounds a bit cheesy." (Volunteer)

> "Generally, our volunteer recruitment comes from other volunteers who have told friends or sometimes it can be service users that have come through and used the service, if it's been beneficial to them and then they decide that they are really appreciative to what we do as an organisation and they want to give something back or just lay people who call and say 'I have seen your organisation, I have seen your website, are you looking for volunteers? I would like to be one'." (Staff)

All volunteers attended an induction day held before they started volunteering where they found out about the core aims and values of the organisation and the range of services provided, met other volunteers, and discussed issues around equal opportunities, confidentiality and boundaries. The induction day was seen to act as a 'bit of a filter', with new volunteers self-selecting activities they wanted to sign up to and ultimately deterring those who were not really committed. Volunteers were then expected to attend training to prepare for their specific role in sexual health outreach, which involved developing awareness of STIs and learning more about ethical issues and confidentiality. In addition, staff tried to get new volunteers to shadow more experienced volunteers or staff.

The investment in the development of both staff and volunteers was a prominent feature of the project and the ethos of the host organisation. The organisation ran 12 training sessions a year, including topics such as listening skills, safer sex, working with vulnerable people and 'coming out' (disclosure of sexuality), and all training sessions were open to both staff and volunteers. Volunteers were expected to attend at least two additional training sessions within the first year of volunteering. Training was seen as a way of giving people the right skills, managing risk and ensuring that volunteers were equipped for work in the community. It meant that volunteers could keep updated with essential information and also that both staff and volunteers could gain further skills that might be useful in their careers.

In general, the sexual health outreach project operated with a core of about eight reliable volunteers. Inevitably, there was some turnover with volunteers leaving because of changes in circumstances, like leaving university or moving jobs. This was accepted not only as inevitable, but also as a driver for investment in training:

> "The sheer amount of training that volunteers have and … because of the turnover rate, it can eat up time and resources. Ideally, we'd love to have loads of long-term volunteers that know everything and only need refresher training once a blue moon but it doesn't work like that. I would say that is the drawback but it is also a positive thing because it keeps us on our toes and makes sure that we are very active in training volunteers." (Staff)

There could at times be a mismatch of expectations between the volunteer role and the social needs of volunteers. One person suggested that some people expected "too much from the role, they were hoping it would cure their loneliness".

The focus on personal development in this case study was reflected in the way volunteers could move into other volunteer roles within the organisation, for example, acting as a trustee for the organisation, administration roles, mentoring or the gay switchboard. The variety of volunteer roles meant that individuals could find something to suit them, thereby putting selection and matching of volunteers firmly in the hands of volunteers themselves. When job vacancies arose within the organisation, volunteers were able to apply for jobs internally. One member of staff stated that there was a preference to recruit internally as volunteers knew how the whole organisation works, and "we know that they have given their time and effort to the service". Social mobility was a key theme, with examples of both individuals progressing on to paid roles and those who were able to enhance their career pathway. The context was markedly different from some of the other case studies, where lay health workers had little formal education or faced barriers to learning.

Equal partners

Across all the People in Public Health case studies, the lay health worker role was valued not just in terms of service capacity, but also in relation to the complementary skills and knowledge brought. In the sexual health outreach project, it was striking that not only were the volunteers, albeit only small in number, integral to the way the project was run, but also that volunteer activity was the bedrock that underpinned how the organisation functioned. The organisational culture was one in which volunteers were regarded as equal partners in a shared enterprise with staff.

This notion of equal worth coexisted with the delivery of screening that was based predominantly on a medical model of disease prevention. In order to deliver those clinical services and satisfy the quality standards demanded by the NHS, clear protocols for the various roles, both professional and lay, were required (see Box 7.1). Volunteers did some of the reception and administration duties connected with the HIV counselling service, but they did not undertake any pre- or post-counselling. They could give out information on screening and could also carry out urine tests in venues where the outreach service was operating but they did not do any vaccinations, as this was the role of sessional nursing staff. A team approach was adopted for the outreach work. Volunteers worked fairly autonomously while on the 'scene' with minimal professional supervision; however, they were encouraged to refer back to staff when complex issues arose or when they were unable to answer questions from clients:

> "We very much class our volunteers as part of the professional team. They are [organisation] staff, so our expectations of our volunteers are incredibly high, but likewise the expectations that somebody will have on the scene, of a[n organisation] volunteer, will be very high. They expect a certain standard from us and part of that is not the service delivered but how it's delivered." (Staff)

Relationships were described in terms of mutual respect and volunteers were valued as essential members of the team. The social aspects of working as a team were highlighted; social activities, both formally arranged and spontaneous, brought people together and were a benefit of volunteering:

> "Yeah very much so, right from, '[Name] we really need you ... you're such a star, thank you!'. And that was the biggest thing for me, I really felt like I was helping them out because they respected my efforts, right from the friendly attitude I got from all the staff ... but that was the main thing, the pat on the back when I agreed to do something, the 'Thank you [name]'." (Volunteer)

> "I've got a core of them [volunteers] who will turn up to anything and do anything and we'll all go out for a drink afterwards and tonight we're packing condoms, so that's quite a sociable bunch so they will come and we'll get some wine or whatever and we'll all go out for a pint afterwards. So there are a core that, a lot of them are my mates, but there is that and some people do, you know, volunteer just to

meet people, which is fair enough, volunteering has many different functions for people." (Staff)

Belonging to the voluntary sector organisation involved accepting a collective identity. Volunteers were literally visible in the community as they wore T-shirts declaring that they were a volunteer, and one volunteer described the recognition that came from working with an organisation that had some credibility in the gay community. Volunteers were seen as ambassadors for the organisation and also a way for the organisation to connect to the community. One member of staff explained that volunteers were used as "our eyes and ears", but also that "it gives the community a good idea of who we are and what we do".

  Belonging brought responsibilities to act in appropriate ways. Trust was a recurrent theme throughout interviews with the different stakeholders, including commissioners and managers. Some of those interviewed described the history of the outreach service and the growing trust placed in volunteers as activities were gradually handed over. One practitioner spoke of how staff had initially been "scared" but that trust had been built up:

> "We were initially going to use volunteers teamed up with a staff member, especially in the community testing side, and the volunteer would shadow and the staff member would do all the talking, but we realised we were giving the volunteers a bit of a disservice and they can be a damn sight brighter than us on a lot of things so why not utilise them and allow them to develop the service…? You don't need a staff member doing it themselves, you don't need a staff member holding their hands." (Staff)

The integration of volunteers in the organisation structure, and the relationship with the wider community, reflects a 'grassroots' rather than 'corporatist' model of voluntary sector organisation (Milligan and Fyfe, 2005). Milligan and Fyfe (2005) found that grassroots organisations were characterised by a non-hierarchical approach to decision-making and that priority was given to active engagement of service users and volunteers, often with a 'club house model' (Milligan and Fyfe, 2005, p 427), with blurring of boundaries between provider and user roles. Certainly, the fact that many of the staff and volunteers had made the journey from being a service user to becoming actively engaged in the organisation may have been an influential factor shaping the organisational ethos and the status of volunteers. Another feature was the way the organisation was embedded in the community and oriented to community needs. Volunteers were seen as performing a vital function of keeping the organisation grounded in the community it served. Overall, the case study illustrates that community connectedness and equality can successfully coexist with the delivery of a clinical health service.

Managing risks

The issue of risk was explored in all the People in Public Health case studies, as risks varied with context and organisations managed risks, particularly those associated with handing over control to community members, in different ways. The sexual health outreach project illustrated the importance of having robust support systems, including training, to underpin lay engagement in delivery. Risks were identified on a number of levels (see Table 7.1). At the most basic level, there were risks associated with handing over the provision of a clinical service to be delivered in non-clinical settings by a non-statutory organisation reliant on volunteers and non-clinical community development workers. The commissioning process meant that it was vital that the service was delivered to acceptable quality standards. Nevertheless, the Primary Care Trust viewed the organisation as 'experts' and allowed them to operate within a broad service-level agreement: "how they actually deliver services is up to them".

In delivering the sexual health outreach services, there were risks associated with peer education and clients receiving correct information. This was largely managed through volunteers accessing a broad training and development programme that enhanced and updated their knowledge and allowed them to reflect on ethical issues such as confidentiality. Volunteers were also encouraged to turn to staff when issues arose that they could not handle and support systems were in place to facilitate that process. There was, however, an acceptance that risks could never be entirely avoided:

> "We try to reduce the risks involved through screening and training, training and training and also refresher training." (Staff)

> "Risks I suppose are ensuring that they are equipped properly with the information to actually go out and deliver it. Touch wood, we haven't had many major issues, but one of the things that we were very aware of was if somebody tried to, and I suppose it's true of the staff team as well, if someone tried to bluster their way through a question instead of just going 'I'll just ask' instead of giving misinformation to that person, which could then affect that person's personal or mental or physical health, so we have to be very aware of that and that the volunteers are shadowed by the staff team and we do review all the time." (Staff)

Risks of lay people complying with professional advice is a concern highlighted in some of the literature (Gaskin, 2006b; Curtis et al, 2007), but little has been written about risks for lay health workers in navigating relationships with their own community. This is perhaps particularly pertinent because the LGBT community have experienced discrimination and exclusion in relation to expressing their sexuality (Daley, 2006). Volunteers in the sexual health project could come across issues through contact with clients that they felt unable to deal with or made them feel distressed. Staff and volunteers had often been on the other side of the fence as service users, and personal experiences could resurface. In addition, working very publically on the 'scene' was not simple. There were occasionally risks to personal safety from 'queer-bashing' and people's reactions to being approached in a social venue were not always predictable. The organisation dealt with it by actively providing support from professional workers and volunteers having access to someone who they could turn to in order to ask questions or for a chance to talk over issues:

> "I think while we're out on the scene we need to be able to reach people in the office should anything come up ... so I think it's important to have a contact person when you're actually working out. It's probably good to have somebody you can talk to afterwards if anything particularly disturbing came up or something you feel you should get some advice on." (Volunteer)

Boundaries between public health work and community life also raised risks around confidentiality. Volunteers and staff could be working on the scene one night and socialising on the scene with their friends the next. This was viewed as an organisational risk and something that was connected to the personal responsibility of volunteers (and staff). The organisation dealt with the risk head on by including discussion of these issues at induction and throughout subsequent

Table 7.1: Risks and risk management with volunteering in sexual health outreach

	Potential risks associated with involving volunteers	Risk management strategies
For volunteer	– Distress from talking to clients. – Personal safety. – Navigating social situations in community.	– Support systems in place in the organisation. – Volunteer coordinator in post. – Volunteers able to turn to project staff for support back at office. – Access to staff when working in bars and clubs.
For organisation	– Breaches of confidentiality. – Clients being given incorrect information.	– Induction to make potential volunteers aware of role and allow people to opt out. – Training for role. – Range of staff development opportunities – all open to volunteers. – Volunteers expected to attend two training sessions every year to keep updated.
For health service	– Arm's length delivery – need to maintain quality standards.	– Protocols with roles clearly defined. – Respecting expertise of voluntary sector organisation.
For community	– Breaches of confidentiality.	– Training on confidentiality given in volunteer induction. – Confidentiality policy in place.

training, and by having a confidentiality policy. Navigating boundaries within social situations, however, required volunteers to have good social skills and self-awareness. One volunteer commented: "You don't go up to them in the gay bar and say 'How was your HIV test last night'", and then went on to say: "it's quite a big ask, it's not just two hours a week. It's constantly being aware of not saying anything you shouldn't".

In summary, risks were present but, overall, these were outweighed by the benefits brought from engaging volunteers in service delivery. Although the emphasis was on enjoyment and personal commitment, the volunteer role came with certain responsibilities that washed over into personal life. The organisation had responsibilities to its clients and to its volunteers and recognition of the risks had shaped the type of support and training provided.

A shared identity?

Swider (2002) raises an important question about whether community health workers need to be peers, in terms of sharing a common identity or being drawn from the same community, or whether the most important characteristics relate to an ability to reach out and empathise with people. Unlike an intervention such as Popular Opinion Leaders (Kelly, 2004), the sexual health project did not have a policy of recruiting people based on their sexuality or standing in the gay community. Some volunteers were heterosexual, although, as some interviewees pointed out, they clearly needed to feel comfortable operating within this community, and, indeed, many of the staff and volunteers identified themselves as gay and had experience as service users.

Common to all the case studies, the pre-eminence of social skills, such as approachability, listening skills, confidence to engage people and empathy, dominated any discussion of qualities. In bars and clubs on the scene, volunteers needed to be outgoing, confident and charismatic, to be able to approach people and engage them in conversation. In some instances, quite high levels of social skills were required, for example, the ability to interpret social situations and make judgements about when to offer information or support and when to hold back when people were drunk or on drugs.

Being 'lay' was considered a critical quality and this meant that volunteers offered something that could not be provided by professional staff (see South et al, 2011a). Barriers could still exist between client and professional, even if that professional was openly gay. One practitioner, for example, spoke of the dangers of "becoming a bit removed from the community" and being in a "work bubble". The lay status of volunteers was contrasted to traditional health services, where men who have sex with men could feel judged. The volunteers were able to offer a more relaxed, informal approach in the bars and clubs and break down barriers to services:

—

"I imagine that there's people that would tell us things just going into a bar they wouldn't tell someone who was dressed like a doctor. So they feel a lot more at ease and also that they aren't being judged and that's the really important thing, because if someone comes up here for an HIV test I don't think they feel like I am making a judgement about their sexual practices whereas if they go to the GUM [Genito-urinary Medicine] clinic some of them would feel that." (Volunteer)

Overall, this case study shows that the mechanisms that supported better links with the community were not dependent on a single set of attributes or being matched peer to peer. The question of identity is therefore one that cannot be resolved simplistically. Non-professional standing, social skills, volunteer (unpaid) status, service user experience and sexuality were all part of the construction of volunteer roles. As is argued elsewhere (South et al, 2011a), lay status, and the agency of the volunteer operating within informal social networks, appeared to be critical to the effectiveness of the programme and volunteers, therefore, brought a distinctive dimension to the sexual health outreach programme. Where volunteers were embedded within their social networks, they were able to cascade information through those networks, but the lay element remained critical:

"And it also has a knock-on effect, so if you train someone so they are more skilled and more aware about their own sexual health as well as being able to talk about it, it's that knock-on effect of them being able to talk to friends and family as well. So any education to do with volunteers around sexual health will only support increased knowledge amongst their own friends as well as what they offer to a project such as [organisation], especially in marginalised groups and target groups." (External partner)

What does this model offer?

The sexual health outreach case study, albeit a small-scale programme, offers a number of pointers to good practice in relation to involving and supporting people in public health roles. One aspect is the investment in the development of people, rather than treating training and support in a purely instrumental way as a means to programme delivery, thus reflecting Shiner's (1999) distinction between 'peer development' and 'peer delivery'. Training and professional support was an investment to aid sustainability and volunteers were able to make personal journeys within the organisation to new roles as well as gain the skills to support engagement. While the inevitable turnover of volunteers caused some frustration, it was also seen as vital and necessary that the organisation was able to draw on lay resources and be able to successfully manage risks.

Box 7.2: Benefits associated with involving volunteers in sexual health outreach

- **Bridging** – volunteers reduce barriers between professionals and the community, as men were more likely to use the service if they see a 'friendly face'.
- **Reach** – volunteers able to reach the community because they were not a clinical professional or an establishment figure. There is also a ripple effect as information flows into the community through natural social networks.
- **Comfort factor** – men who have sex with men are not being judged.
- **Capacity** – leaves professionals free to do other things.
- **Community knowledge** – knowledge can feed in from the community to the organisation. Volunteers are the 'eyes and ears' of the organisation; this also raises the organisational profile in the community.
- **Personal gains** – volunteers experience personal satisfaction and enjoyment, as well as enhanced career prospects.

Source: Adapted from South et al (2011a, p 308).

The case study provides good evidence of the nature and value of the lay contribution as a strategy to address health inequalities in this community and a number of benefits were identified (see Box 7.2). Undoubtedly, the inclusion of volunteers enhanced the programme's effectiveness and increased its reach, but this was not about quasi-professionals helping an overstretched service. Like the Walking for Health case study in Chapter Six, what appears to be a very simple model of volunteers in a defined role – here, increasing uptake of screening – in fact consists of complex processes building relationships between voluntary organisation, volunteers and the community. The wider effects of these processes, particularly in relation to supporting improved connections with the community and the bilateral flow of information, provide a powerful illustration of the potential of the bridging role to lead to redesigned services more in tune with community needs:

> "I think it's really important, that ethos sort of with not just the [project] but the whole organisation about volunteers is that they do form that fundamental part of the organisation, that is not the organisation or the service user it's sort of more that bit in between. They are much more closer to the service user and service users will probably more identify with volunteers as opposed to a staff member who is getting paid to do that. So, more often than not, they will come from the community that we serve and, more often than not, our volunteers come from our communities and therefore have that first-hand knowledge of what ... kind of services are needed and that is very much fed into the whole ethos organisation that we provide." (Staff)

Key points

- This case study highlights the use of peer-based approaches to raise awareness of sexual health and improve access to screening. Volunteers were able to reach out to a community who faced barriers to using traditional health services.
- Volunteers were integral to the way the organisation worked and helped the organisation maintain good connections with the community.
- The risks of involving volunteers were managed through investing in the personal development of volunteers, offering induction and training, having clear protocols, and ensuring volunteers had access to support when needed.
- Volunteers were valued as equal partners, and the case study shows that an inclusive, community-oriented culture can successfully coexist with the delivery of a clinical outreach service.

EIGHT

Community Health Educators – a case study

One of the primary motivations for involving lay people in delivering health promotion activities is the potential to engage underserved or marginalised populations who experience poor health. This chapter presents findings from a case study of a Community Health Educators programme, where the lay health workers performed a bridging role within disadvantaged urban neighbourhoods, taking out health messages to local communities and supporting people to participate in healthy activities. The Community Health Educators were recruited from the communities they worked with and the programme focused on their personal development and empowerment. The case study is of interest because the programme pursued an inclusive, flexible approach to recruitment, training and supervision, including using sessional payment to support the Community Health Educators in their work. The chapter highlights some of the tensions arising between empowerment approaches and having to deliver against health targets, as well discussing the thorny issue of payment versus volunteering. The chapter starts by looking at the Community Health Educator model and how it relates to other roles more common in international contexts, such as Lay Health Advisors. It then goes on to look at the Community Health Educators programme as a strategy for tackling inequalities, prior to discussing some of the dilemmas in practice.

Background

The Community Health Educator model first emerged in the UK in the 1990s, with innovative programmes such as Woman-to-Woman: Promoting Cervical Screening to Minority Ethnic Women in Primary Care (1994–97) and Straight Talking: Communicating Breast Screening Messages in Primary Care (2000–02) (Chiu, 2003). Chiu, who played a key role in the development of these programmes, describes the Community Health Educator model as based on the twin principles of empowerment and participation, drawing heavily on the radical ideas of Paulo Freire (1970):

> Community Health Educators are members of the community who are trusted by community members, and they take on the role of consciousness awareness-raising through facilitating discussion and critical questioning of issues that concern the community. (Chiu, 2003, p 3)

Initially, the model was developed working with minority ethnic women, but was later applied in other communities experiencing disadvantage. Community members typically undertake an in-depth training course that not only educates them about relevant health issues and develops their communication and organisational skills, but also develops their critical awareness and ability to reflect on community health needs (Chiu, 2003). There are currently a number of Community Health Educator programmes across the UK. For example, in Sheffield, a consortium of community and voluntary organisations provides training and support to a network of over 200 volunteer community health champions who develop and deliver health activities in some of the most disadvantaged communities in Sheffield (Sheffield Well-being Consortium, no date[a]). For a case story of one of the champions, see Chapter Five.

The Community Health Educator model is predicated on lay health workers being able to use their personal networks and their 'social embeddedness' within communities to reach out to groups not in touch with services (Chiu and West, 2007). The model shares much in common with Lay Health Advisor programmes in the US, where the emphasis is on bridging roles as a strategy to tackle health inequalities, particularly around access to health care (Eng et al, 1997; Jackson and Parks, 1997). There is some evidence that these programmes have been successful at increasing uptake of screening (Lam et al, 2003), and in adoption of positive health behaviours (Fleury et al, 2009). Rhodes et al (2007) identify the assumptions that underpin the approach: that Lay Health Advisors are part of the target community, have an understanding of social networks, communicate in a common language and are able to incorporate cultural practice into their health promotion activities. Jackson and Parks (1997) reiterate that 'true' Lay Health Advisors are individuals who are identified by the community as being natural helpers; however, their review of practice uncovered many examples where recruitment was based on professional judgement. In a UK study of Community Health Educators' social networks, Chiu and West (2007, p 1925) concluded that reliance on a high degree of embeddedness 'may yield little effective connectivity' and that Community Health Educators need both to utilise their 'strong ties' within personal networks and to cultivate 'weak ties' with local organisations.

Community Health Educators – a case study

The Community Health Educators programme was chosen as a case study for the People in Public Health study because the engagement of lay health workers in addressing health inequalities represented an example of the bridging model and because the use of sessional payment provided a contrast to the projects based on volunteering. The Community Health Educator programme was delivered through a voluntary sector organisation operating as a healthy living network, which coordinated a number of health projects across the city and had been established as part of the Healthy Living Centre initiative (Hills et al, 2007). The Community Health Educator programme, which was a core part of the work of the healthy living network, involved training local people, who undertook a 14-week accredited course in preparation for carrying out health promotion activities in their communities. Once trained, Community Health Educators were supported through the network to deliver or assist in the delivery of group sessions or community events, with a focus on communicating simple, preventive health messages. The programme worked with a wide range of population groups, including geographic communities, mostly in disadvantaged neighbourhoods, minority ethnic populations and marginalised groups (see Table 8.1). Many of the activities involved Community Health Educators working with professionals in various settings, including schools, prisons and residential homes. As well as the generic programme, the healthy living network trained Community Health Educators for two specific health projects; one promoting access to affordable fruit and vegetables in some of the city's most disadvantaged communities; and the other promoting a healthy and active life with older people at risk of social isolation.

Initially, the programme was funded through the New Opportunities Fund, but later there was a shift to a city-wide network to broaden potential funding sources. At the time of the case study, there was a mix of service-level agreements with statutory organisations, the local Primary Care Trust being a major commissioner, whereas the two specified health projects described earlier were commissioned through a regional health and well-being programme.

The Community Health Educator programme was explicitly underpinned by community development principles in that it sought to build community capacity through developing the skills and confidence of individuals to enable them to work with fellow community members in an empowering way. One of the programme documents stated: 'We are all about local people in areas of high need taking back control and having increased power over their health'. Although some activities were based on peer education methods, the programme was flexible in its approach and had the capacity to support communities organising to address locally identified needs. A total of 21 interviews were conducted as part of the case study. Ten members of staff involved in managing or delivering the programme were interviewed, including tutors and community development

Table 8.1: Community Health Educators – what they do and who they work with

Groups – examples	Settings – examples	Health topics – examples	Partners – examples
– Gypsies and Travellers	– Community centres	– Diabetes	– Community groups
– Older people	– Community events	– Drug misuse	– Occupational
– People who misuse	and festivals	– Healthy eating	therapists
drugs	– Churches, mosques	– Cardiovascular	– Residential home staff
– People with learning	and temples	disease prevention	– Teachers and school
disabilities	– Prisons and Young	– Mental health	leaders
– Prisoners' families	Offender Institutions	– Physical activity	
– Schoolchildren	– Residential and care	– Sexual health	
– Women's groups	homes	– Smoking cessation	
	– Schools	– Stress and relaxation	
	– Traveller camps		

workers, and two external partners with commissioning roles. Nine Community Health Educators were interviewed, four of these were working with the older people's project. It was not possible to interview any service users because many of the activities involved only brief interactions.

Bridging roles – a strategy for tackling health inequalities

The rationale behind the Community Health Educators programme was to involve people from disadvantaged neighbourhoods and groups to undertake health promotion activities in their communities, thereby acting as 'connectors' in much the same way as the Lay Health Advisor model (Eng et al, 1997; Rhodes et al, 2007). Community Health Educators could, it was argued, "cover more ground" making additional contacts to health professionals and, moreover, provide that vital bridge between health services and communities: "The reason they're there is that they are the absolute interface between hard-to- reach, vulnerable, isolated [groups] and other preventative work" (external partner).

The programme emphasised both *scale*, with around 59 Community Health Educators active at the time of the case study, and *reach*, working with disadvantaged or excluded groups who might experience barriers to accessing preventive services (see Table 8.1). The focus was on what one practitioner described as "fast and rapid engagement", an "industrialisation" strategy to bring about behaviour change. There was an explicit strategy to recruit people from the target groups and to maintain an inclusive view of what individuals could contribute. The journeys of Community Health Educators were part of capacity-building, as people gained in confidence and self-esteem, developed employable skills and sometimes moved into employment. Health inequalities were, therefore, being addressed by the programme in three ways:

- through the personal development of people who were drawn from disadvantaged groups or neighbourhoods;
- through their subsequent role in engaging groups who were at risk of poor health; and
- through building capacity to address locally identified needs via these routes of engagement.

The value of recruiting individuals from less advantaged communities was that they could empathise and connect with people with whom they shared similar experiences. Being of equal social standing was important. One community health educator said: "we're just normal people, aren't we, and they can relate to us"; while another reflected that having similar experiences made it easier for people to approach them. A number of those we interviewed spoke of the existing barriers between communities and health professionals and the role of Community Health Educators in breaking down those barriers because of their ability to access social networks and their approachability:

"It allows you to interact with community members who would never in a million years go near the NHS or any other professional service, and in extreme cases have an absolute pathological hatred of authority." (Staff)

"The people are from the heart of communities, so they'll experience all the problems that that community experience so that they've got an inner knowledge and they've often got a trust within a community that a professional won't have." (Staff)

Several Community Health Educators were able to speak more than one language, and, in some cases, English was their second language. Such language skills enabled the programme to access minority ethnic communities. For example, one Community Health Educator worked with Chinese elders to set up an exercise class and then supported participation, including offering interpretation.

Box 8.1 provides some examples of activities undertaken by Community Health Educators, which illustrate the ways that engagement processes worked to support health goals and potentially reduce inequalities. Much of the work could be described as low-intensity health education, in that the primary purpose of many group activities was to convey simple health messages, yet Community Health Educators were able to raise awareness of health issues informally using methods that people could engage with. The approach was most often participatory and aimed to be inclusive, with those attending group activities able to contribute their own knowledge or make suggestions for further activities. The benefits were seen to include strengthening individuals' sense of self-esteem, breaking down barriers within a community, increasing opportunities for interaction and reducing social isolation. Being embedded in the community also brought benefits. There were cases of Community Health Educators proactively responding to identified community needs, or acting as role models in their community, with other residents picking up messages from their behaviour:

"Because we've gone back into our community, the community know who we are and they've seen some of the work that we've done, they do come back to us all: 'Could you put this on for us?', or 'How do you go about?', or 'Can you support us?'. And we're signposting them as well, as we know our area quite well now." (Community Health Educator)

Box 8.1: Connecting with communities

Community Health Educators attended community events, such as fetes, providing free tasters of fruit presented as fruit kebabs or smoothies. One Community Health Educator described doing a session in a class at school:"I did a quiz at the end of it and they reeled it off and I were like gob-smacked of how much information they had just absorbed from what I'd given them".

The healthy living network organised an event so that older people could have their flu jabs at a community centre rather than attending their general practice. At this event, described as more like "going to a social event rather than just walking into a doctor's surgery", health professionals were able to immunise large numbers of residents in one session, while Community Health Educators talked to people informally about health issues as they waited.

Community Health Educators ran a series of healthy eating classes to develop the cookery skills of a cohort of school students. They subsequently organised sessions in a sheltered housing complex, where the students shared newly developed skills with a group of older people, who were also able to share some of their experiences with the students. The success of this joint learning approach was evidenced by the change in attitude of the students, and benefits were seen to be as much about community cohesion as healthy eating.

A 'sloppy slippers' campaign was run in care homes and sheltered housing where Community Health Educators worked with the podiatrists in assessing the suitability of older people's footwear, and swapping their old slippers for better-fitting, safer items. Community Health Educators engaged in informal conversations with residents, offering information and advice on a wide range of health issues, as well as referring people on to health professionals if required.

As a strategy for addressing health inequalities, the engagement of lay health workers who are drawn from and work with disadvantaged communities has implications for programme delivery and management. This case study illustrates the need for supportive processes to be in place to enable individuals to adopt a bridging role. Three themes emerging from the case study are now discussed: adopting an inclusive approach to involvement; empowerment through training and personal development; and offering a flexible work structure supported by remuneration.

Valuing life experience

The philosophy of the Community Health Educators programme, in line with community development principles, is about valuing individuals as community assets and seeking to build their capacity to contribute to the health agenda. Like the other case study projects, individuals' life experience and pre-existing skills were regarded as vital attributes in helping to connect with communities and carry out the lay health worker role. This contrasts to what might be termed deficit models, where lay health workers are defined by a lack of professional skills, which are regarded as implicitly of a higher order (see, eg, Public Health Resource Unit and Skills for Health, 2008).

In terms of the skills and characteristics required, there was a consensus across both lay and professional stakeholders. Interest in the community was considered crucial to the Community Health Educator role and altruism, a desire to contribute to the community, was found to be the main motivating factor. Indeed, some of the Community Health Educators brought previous voluntary experience and the role was seen as extending their capabilities to address community needs. Local knowledge, knowing "what the community has, what the community needs, what kind of people are living in that community", and lived experience were seen as critical in reaching out to target communities:

> "If you want an ex-offender to come on [a] CHE course, who better to send to chat to them than an ex-offender with a criminal record, or who better to explain a detox process to another alcoholic [than someone who] is a recovering alcoholic." (Staff)

Like the other case studies, communication, organisational and social skills were emphasised and were also identified in the job specification (see Table 8.2). Community Health Educators were expected to be able to communicate with a wide range of people, but this was not solely about delivering health messages. It also concerned the ability to engage other community members in an approachable and informal manner, as one Community Health Educator described: "I can go into a group of women that are stood nattering away and I can sort of squeeze myself in and say 'Excuse me', and just get myself involved" (Community Health Educator). A further set of attributes that was seen as significant, in the context of working with clients from vulnerable groups, concerned the ability of Community Health Educators to act respectfully and sensitively towards the people they were working with.

Discussions on motivations and skills focused on personal development: building skills, capacities and confidence. One Community Health Educator captured this ethos succinctly, observing: "I think anybody can be what they want to be, if they're shown the way or if they're given a bit of support and the opportunity". Notwithstanding the benefits of an inclusive approach, there are evidently implications for the type of training and support offered, as the programme needed to be able to bring capabilities to the fore, whatever an individual's starting point.

Table 8.2: Community Health Educators – person specification

Skills	Attitude
– Good communication skills in English or possibly another community language	– Commitment to the concept of Community Health Educators
– Ability to record and report	– Ability to work in a supportive manner
– One-to-one or group-working skills	– Willingness to work flexibly and to travel around the area
– Basic organisational abilities	– Willingness to learn new material and topics on health matters
– Understanding issues around confidentiality	
– Listening and advocacy skills	
– Cultural and religious sensitivity	
– Problem-solving and decision-making	

Empowering people

One of the building blocks for personal development was the 14-week Community Health Educator course run through the healthy living network to cohorts of around 15 participants who attended for one day a week. The course was accredited with the Open College Network and participants could opt to obtain either an NVQ level 2 qualification or, if they were prepared to submit some additional written work, an NVQ level 3. The course aimed to raise awareness of health issues and prepare Community Health Educators to work with their communities and included units on 'Power and powerlessness' and 'Building strengths in communities'. Optional units, such as drug/alcohol awareness, were included depending on the skills and interests of each cohort. As well as the initial training, Community Health Educators were given opportunities to access additional courses to equip them to carry out their role, for example, basic food hygiene training, conflict resolution or walk leadership. Where appropriate, some of these courses were accredited, so that individuals were able to add to their portfolio of qualifications.

There was strong evidence that participation in the programme, including the initial training, had a significant impact on the confidence and skills of those involved. Self-esteem, confidence, employability and improvements in mental health were all identified as significant outcomes: "The big gain is in people having a fairly intensive input that's quite creative and allows them to develop themselves and their skills" (external partner).

There was a sense of mutual support between participants, which often continued after the initial training. The training could also be a way of validating prior knowledge and experiences. One Community Health Educator, for example, claimed that as well as providing "the tools to go back out into the community and to do whatever we can", the training had helped her realise that "you have no idea how many skills you have, you know, the things that you do in normal daily life are actually incredibly important". Others described how the training and working with people from other communities broadened their understanding of different health and social issues.

Personal development and empowerment was also supported through practice. Community Health Educators reportedly grew in confidence as they tried activities and became aware that they were effective communicators. This might lead, in turn, to taking opportunities to progress in new directions:

> "It's built up my confidence as well ... it builds up your confidence and you're able to go and work, go off and do other things and it helps people come off the benefits and go into jobs and things." (Community Health Educator)

There was a clear commitment across the programme to provide the necessary support to keep Community Health Educators engaged and to enable them to achieve personal goals. The challenge was that people's starting points and their subsequent journeys were very different. While some Community Health Educators progressed quickly within the role to start to design and deliver community activities independently, others required supervision for some considerable time after their training. One practitioner cautioned that:

> "Although CHEs [Community Health Educators] are trained up to OCN [Open College Network] level 2 or 3, it gives them maybe enough confidence to start off, you know, go out into the community and passing on health messages, but it doesn't make them a fully fledged health promotion warrior." (Staff)

There was evidence that participation in the programme could be a springboard to other roles or, alternatively, deeper levels of engagement within the community. Some individuals were motivated to undertake training because they saw it as a way to prepare for entering the job market after a period of worklessness. Becoming a Community Health Educator could be a mechanism to achieve personal goals. Examples of progression included: moving to paid employment as a project worker in the healthy living network; becoming a health trainer; establishing a holistic health consultancy; and developing new services within a carer support network.

Flexibility and payment

Like many community projects, the Community Health Educators programme needed to achieve a balance between meeting the support needs of individual lay health workers and meeting the health needs of the community. A distinctive challenge here, resulting from the inclusive approach adopted for recruitment and training, was the wide variation in the competencies, experiences and capacities of individual Community Health Educators. Two defining features of the support systems established in this case study were a flexible approach to working patterns and the use of sessional payment.

Community Health Educators were free to opt in to as much or as little activity as they wanted, both in terms of number and frequency of sessions and in relation to the intensity of the role. This flexibility around work patterns is more often associated with volunteer rather than paid roles. However, many of the Community Health Educators had other commitments, including other voluntary or paid work or caring responsibilities, and the flexibility allowed them to juggle the different elements of their lives: "The thing that appealed to me most, even more than the money, was the fact that it was sessional … I could pick and choose … I wasn't committed to anything and tied down to anything" (Community Health Educator).

While flexibility might be seen to support engagement, it presented challenges to programme managers: first, in terms of equity where people were taking very different levels of responsibility but receiving the same pay; and, second, in terms of ensuring that there were sufficient Community Health Educators able to carry out health activities independently.

Community Health Educators received payment for sessions worked, based on an hourly payment rate that varied according to what project they were working on. The hourly rates in 2009 when the research was conducted ranged from £7 to £9, with a £1.40 per hour holiday pay. Despite some of these challenges, the provision of remuneration, in the context of social and economic disadvantage, was viewed positively as a factor supporting engagement, particularly by the Community Health Educators themselves. These findings are supported by other research which suggests that remuneration is a key factor aiding retention; however, it is undoubtedly a complex issue (Leaman et al, 1997; Taylor et al, 2001; Lehmann and Sanders, 2007). For some Community Health Educators, receiving payment gave them a sense of worth and was seen as recognition of their contribution: "it's like being valued, being given that little bit of money is just like being valued". For others, economic need meant that it was essential to receive some payment to support their engagement: "I think it is [important], I have to survive, it's important that I have something to take away".

For those on welfare benefits, payment might be a welcome injection of income, but benefits rules were problematic. There were examples of how Community Health Educators had been unable to deliver activities for fear of having benefits reduced or stopped. On the other hand, the flexible work structure afforded individuals the opportunity to work within the rules (albeit for as little as two hours a week), and that was seen to help boost job prospects. Payment could be a way of putting money back into local communities, delivering economic along with social benefits in line with some of the features of Intermediate Labour Market programmes (Finn and Simmonds, 2003).

There were some disadvantages to the programme's approach to financial support, although these were given much less prominence in the interviews. Payment could potentially exclude volunteers or undermine the volunteer ethos, but, interestingly, there was no evidence that it undermined the altruistic response of Community Health Educators to serve their communities. One dilemma was that inequities could emerge in a pay system that gave equal reward to Community Health Educators who had varying capabilities and were taking on different levels of responsibility. Remuneration brought additional costs and, therefore, was a potential threat to sustainability.

Tensions between empowerment approaches and the health system

The case study provided an opportunity to understand better the frictions that can occur between empowerment approaches and the pursuit of public health priorities. The principles of empowerment approaches involve a shift away from professional power towards people taking greater control of their lives and health (Rappaport, 1987; Wallerstein, 1992). The logic of this approach is that programmes are there in an enabling role, to support and guide where required, but not to direct or limit action. This was the stance of the project staff in supporting the personal development and empowerment of participants recruited to the Community Health Educator course. Independent community action may, however, as this case study illustrates, sometimes be in conflict with professional priorities dominant in the health system.

Notwithstanding the success of the programme in terms of engaging local people in public health, there were tensions between the personal development of the Community Health Educators and the need to respond to health service priorities, where there was seen to be an increasing push, through the commissioning process, to demonstrate impact on the target communities. For example, due to the pressure to achieve specified health-related outcomes, one of the projects had begun to take a more selective approach to recruitment to ensure that Community Health Educators were able operate independently following training. While the Community Health Educators programme was seen to be successful in terms of reach – getting to communities and groups that were not necessarily in touch with mainstream services – there were questions raised about the effectiveness of low-intensity brief interventions, where large numbers of contacts were generated but with little evidence of behaviour change in the short term. At the same time, there was recognition from all stakeholder groups that the programme had a transformative effect on many Community Health Educators and was having an impact through social networks. The paradox was that the ability of empowered lay workers to connect was of value to health services but this made it difficult to control or to capture effects.

The Community Health Educators programme was independent of the NHS yet received funding through it to undertake health promotion activities. While accredited training, supervision and reporting systems to funders all contributed to quality assurance, the programme did not, and, indeed, could not, prevent Community Health Educators going 'off message' or going beyond the boundaries of the role. Although the risks of using an approach where Community Health Educators were empowered rather than controlled were discussed by practitioners, there was no evidence that this was a major problem in delivering activities. However, it was reported that health professionals sometimes inadvertently undermined Community Health Educators by highlighting their low level of qualifications:

> "Sometimes people have been to groups and said that they've come back and felt like they were a bit stupid just because they hadn't got the qualifications that other people assumed … because I think people sometimes assume, if you're working in health, you must be trained formally as some kind of health practitioner." (Staff)

Recruiting local residents allowed health services to connect with communities, but that was no guarantee of smooth relationships. In the interviews, several respondents spoke of how Community Health Educators did not always behave in line with recognised 'work etiquette' and sometimes communication with professionals broke down. Ultimately, the empowerment approach enabled individuals to make a contribution, who in other contexts would have been excluded from provider roles, but did not produce compliant lay health workers. Indeed, the programme training was designed to raise critical consciousness about community needs and to foster individual confidence to enact change. As one practitioner explained: "they don't fit into a nice professionalised world, they won't be deferential to any hierarchical system here". Given some of the tensions described, the case study illustrates that a balance has to be struck between the risks of allowing creativity and independence and the risks of inappropriate professionalisation of lay health workers:

> "As soon as we have to sort of regimentalise it, it gets a bit dead. The better qualified they are, the more likely it is that what comes out is a bit sanitised ... the key thing that's happening is that somebody is engaging, then we can trust them to say the right things. We want people who are enthusiastic, and who understand the local picture, it may not need to be 100% accurate, as long as it's fairly accurate." (External partner)

What can this model offer?

The Community Health Educators programme shares similarities with Lay Health Advisor models, because it involves lay health workers in embedded community activity where they rely on their cultural competence to translate health messages and provide a conduit for health services to reach underserved communities (Rhodes et al, 2007). This case study illustrates the potential for these models as a strategy for tackling health inequalities, as Community Health Educators were highly successful in accessing communities that for one reason or another were disengaged from health services. There are questions, some of which were raised during the interviews, about the extent to which this type of rapid, mass engagement can be expected to deliver behavioural outcomes at a population level. Other indicators of success, therefore, such as increased social capital, may offer more appropriate measures of effectiveness.

In terms of service delivery matters, the case study demonstrates that an inclusive approach to recruitment, training and support can lead to individuals gaining confidence and capacity to work in these roles. There was evidence that sessional payment supported engagement in this context. The issue of payment is complex because it touches on matters of fairness and value. Additionally, the boundaries between volunteering and low-paid work may be blurred in areas of high worklessness (Baines and Hardill, 2008). There are real choices over remuneration, particularly where communities experience material disadvantage, but the issue needs active management, not least because of the welfare benefits rules. This topic is discussed further in Chapter Ten.

Finally, this chapter provides an example of how empowerment approaches can work in practice. Although operating in very different contexts, both the sexual health outreach project (Chapter Seven) and the Community Health Educators programme shared the same focus on personal development and progression. Community Health Educators articulated a growing confidence forged initially through the training and later through carrying out the role. The empowerment of cohorts of people, largely drawn from disadvantaged communities, can be seen as a real achievement and one that ultimately may have a greater impact than the low-intensity activities they engage in. Chiu (2003) argues that the benefits of using a Community Health Educator model are threefold: the community development potential; the organisational development potential, as more culturally sensitive services emerge; and the personal development potential in terms of community leadership. This case study illustrates that these types of projects are best understood in terms of investment in the development of individuals who can not only act as connectors, but also initiate processes of long-term change within their communities.

Key points

- This case study offers a UK example of lay health workers in a bridging role. Community Health Educators, largely drawn from disadvantaged groups or neighbourhoods, were successful in reaching out to and engaging with groups who were at risk of poor health.
- The programme adopted an empowerment approach, focusing on the personal development of individuals and equipping them with the confidence and skills to address community needs.
- There was an inclusive approach to recruiting and supporting people with varying needs and abilities to become Community Health Educators. Sessional payment and flexible working patterns were key factors in supporting engagement.
- There can be tensions between empowerment approaches and professional culture, but this case study shows that being identified with the community and having access to social networks were critical to the success of the model.

NINE

Citizen involvement in neighbourhood health – a case study

Community health projects come in all shapes and sizes; some work with a particular community of interest or a specific health theme, others are more generic, delivering a range of health promotion activities often in a neighbourhood setting or based within a community centre. Such projects have been part of the landscape of health promotion in the UK since the 1970s (Tones and Tilford, 2001; Amos, 2002); nonetheless, projects are often small-scale, overly reliant on funding from short-term grants and rarely incorporated into mainstream health provision. The case study presented in this chapter provides a critical examination of volunteering within a small neighbourhood health project based on a disadvantaged housing estate. High levels of community participation were sought and volunteer activity was linked to a community committee involved in the development of health activities on the estate. The chapter looks at the practical challenges and benefits resulting from a deep level of citizen involvement and provides some insights into the dilemmas of achieving sustainability when responsibilities are handed to volunteer workers embedded within their community. The chapter starts with a brief background section summarising approaches to community-based health promotion.

Community-based health promotion

Community participation is a central feature of community health projects, which Tones and Tilford (2001) define as projects that use community development strategies in order to address health issues. Community development broadly concerns community empowerment and collective action to tackle social injustice and build healthy communities (Barr and Hashagen, 2000; Ledwith, 2005). Whitehead (2007) identifies strengthening communities by building mutual support and social inclusion as a category of actions to tackle health inequalities. There has been a long tradition of community health projects in the UK, mostly based within disadvantaged neighbourhoods, stretching back to the Peckham experiment in the 1930s. The New Labour government gave emphasis to area-based initiatives in regeneration and health that sought community involvement in planning and implementation, and many community health projects were developed through initiatives such as Health Action Zones (Bauld and Judge, 2002) and the Healthy Living Centre initiative (Hills et al, 2007). Notwithstanding these policy drivers for greater citizen involvement, Bridgen (2004) cautions that assumptions should not be made that all community-based health schemes use empowerment approaches or seek to extend community influence.

In considering lay health worker roles within community health projects, community members will often carry out a variety of roles, ranging from participation in steering groups through to organising community events, running community cafes and helping with group and outreach activities. The holistic, collective approach means that flexibility is required and roles are not necessarily well defined. Banks (2003) proposes the term 'community practice' to encompass both paid community workers and volunteers because, she argues, practice at neighbourhood level is often underpinned by common values and the broad goal of supporting community activity. The People in Public Health scoping study identified a community organising model where lay health workers play a significant role in the mobilisation of community resources (South et al, 2010b). The North Carolina Breast Cancer Screening Program, for example, involved multi-level programme activity, including locality development to build community capacity, local leadership and volunteer outreach networks (Altpeter et al, 1998). Professional community workers acted as coaches and provided opportunities for training and skills development in order to support community members' efforts at organising themselves.

Expectations about the role of community members and the degree of community control, reflect broad theoretical divisions between what Morgan (2001, p 221) terms 'utilitarian models', where community resources, including labour, are used as a means to deliver a project, and empowerment approaches, where the community members become involved in developing their own solutions to problems. NICE guidance on community engagement suggests that interventions with higher levels of community control can be expected to have a greater impact on health with positive outcomes at an individual and societal level (National Institute for Health and Clinical Excellence, 2008, p 8).

Community participation in a neighbourhood health project – a case study

The neighbourhood health project was set up in 2002 with the aim of improving the health of local residents on a large urban estate. The project was initially funded through the New Deal for Communities, an area-based regeneration programme established by the New Labour government (Neighbourhood Renewal Unit, 2003), and the neighbourhood health project was part of a portfolio of regeneration activities on the estate themed around employment, health, education, crime and the living environment. When the research was undertaken, the project was being delivered through a partnership between the 10-year New Deal for Communities programme, the local authority, which met some staffing costs and provided support, and the local Primary Care Trust, which commissioned some health promotion activities. The project operated from a building in a small shopping centre on the estate and offered residents a place to seek advice, to join one of the organised groups or to access information about other services available in the area. Project activities focused on improving health inequalities in the area through addressing lifestyle issues such as poor diet, smoking and lack of exercise. Examples included:

- a drop-in session with information about health and well-being matters;
- a weekly health walk with a group of local people;
- Tai Chi classes;
- Weightbusters – a weigh-in and discussion for people concerned about their weight;
- smoking cessation sessions with support, advice and information available, delivered in partnership with the Primary Care Trust; and
- events, such as picnics, and trips away from the estate.

The neighbourhood health project employed only two project workers, a community health development officer and part-time administrator, and was therefore reliant on a small cohort of volunteers, mainly local residents, to help run the health promotion activities offered. Volunteer roles in the project were diverse, with volunteers providing assistance to paid staff, collecting money and keeping registers, staffing stalls at community events, providing smoking cessation advice alongside health professionals, signposting to local services, and providing support and advice about health–related issues such as weight loss. Volunteers also independently ran a social group for isolated people with mobility problems at the project, where they provided refreshments, organised games and activities, and offered support while providing a place for residents to socialise and discuss any problems.

The neighbourhood health project was selected as a case study because it offered an example of the community organising model, with its explicit aims to build capacity within the community and to empower residents to improve their own health. Volunteering in the project was linked to an independent community health committee consisting of a small group of residents who were actively involved with the project. This committee aimed to help local residents obtain healthier lifestyles by the active promotion of exercise and healthy eating and to provide a mechanism for community participation into planning processes. There was a reciprocal relationship between the neighbourhood health project and the community health committee, as most of the eight committee members were actively volunteering in the project and, at the same time, the committee received some organisational support from the project to develop health promotion activities on the estate. The committee had successfully bid for money from a Primary Care Trust to establish the social group that volunteers ran independently. It was hoped that the committee would eventually be able to generate an income and become self-sustaining when regeneration monies ended. In conducting the case study, the research team were able to visit the project and observe project activities first hand. Interviews were conducted with 14 individuals; six volunteers (all but one were also members of the community health committee); four staff involved in the management or delivery of the project; and four external partners working at a strategic level. Fifteen individuals attending project activities as service users were also interviewed.

Handing over control

Like many area-based programmes, the New Deal regeneration programme in the estate reflected New Labour policy of encouraging greater community involvement in service planning and delivery and supporting communities to generate their own solutions to social and health problems (Department of Health, 2003; Carr et al, 2006; Sullivan et al, 2006). These aspirations threaded through the discourse around participation in the neighbourhood health project and were enacted in three ways: through the establishment of the community health committee as part of the regeneration programme; by the explicit goal of community-led health activity to become self-managed and self-sustaining; and in the centrality of volunteer involvement to the delivery of project activities.

Both staff involved in project delivery and those working at a strategic level emphasised the underpinning community development principles and the ultimate goal of handing over control to the community to achieve sustainability. One strategic lead reflected on the "high expectations" in the regeneration programme that "somehow ... the power and resources could transfer to a community group". Another stated that volunteers were "one of the keys to sustaining the project because we sort of rely on them to actually keep it going when the [regeneration] funding has ended".

The argument was advanced that community participation enabled the project to fit better with community needs. This rationale was based on recognition of the importance of being in touch with a community and allowing community views to shape the project. Local knowledge meant that "it's more relevant for a community, rather than something that a professional's dreamed up that they think people need". Furthermore, volunteer involvement enabled the project to access the community and cascade messages about health promotion activities on offer. One individual summarised the various justifications:

> "For the model we put forward as part of our bid always involved using residents and volunteers to help us carry out the work because, one, we thought it was ... the way forward really in terms of sustainability, but also because we believe in that community development and involvement approach as being more effective, particularly you know if you're working in a community in a locality because that's how people operate really. One, they're well placed to network if you get involved with, you know, the right kind of people. Two, it's good to hear where they're coming from and how things are, just for people living in a locality because you can make all sorts of assumptions but

if you don't really live there you don't really know. So it's always good to get views of people and feedback as you're developing things … but they're also really good advocates for things and they'll go out and spread the word." (Staff)

With only two project workers, the small cohort of volunteers provided essential support for the delivery of health promotion activities and many worked long hours at the project. Most of the volunteers were actively engaged in democratic processes in the community health committee. Much of the volunteer contribution in the project involved supporting group activities, typically setting up and clearing away, collecting money, providing refreshments, and supporting participants in exercise classes or walks. Some volunteers were involved in providing peer support as a part of a community-based smoking cessation service.

Overall, the lay contribution was critical to the delivery of health improvement activities through the project. Many interviewees commented that the project simply would not exist without the efforts of the volunteers. Community members attending the project recognised the level of commitment demonstrated by volunteers, while, more controversially, a practitioner said that "they are working, they're just unpaid workers … they have very similar training to myself".

Giving and gaining

The rationale for community involvement advanced from a professional perspective focused on the wider goals of the regeneration programme. In contrast, from a lay perspective, volunteers described their engagement in terms of a contribution to their community (giving back) and the personal gains and achievements that reinforced their involvement. All the volunteers were local residents or lived in the surrounding neighbourhoods, many having lived all their lives on the estate, raising their families there. Altruism was a primary motivating factor and volunteers expressed pride in their neighbourhood, combined with a passion for the work that they were doing. It was acknowledged that a strong sense of community inspired some to be involved: "And I'm not doing it because I've got the time, I'm doing it because it's for the community I live in" (volunteer).

The personal benefits from being involved provided a further motivation. Most of the volunteers had long-standing health conditions and volunteering in the project brought enjoyment, mental stimulation and the opportunity to socialise. Some reported feeling lonely and isolated before they became involved in the project, or joining because they were at a loose end.

The dual nature of the contribution, both gaining from involvement and giving back, appeared to strengthen participation. High levels of commitment to the project and to the wider community were in evidence, and there were positive benefits to individuals resulting from that engagement. As discussed in Chapter Five, volunteering was rewarding and could lead to a sense of achievement as others gained through project activities. Furthermore, volunteers were appreciated by project workers and were made to feel valued partners in the shared enterprise of the project. Social aspects of volunteering led to new friendships, and wider personal networks: "Being a volunteer you feel like you belong, well, within this group anyway. They're a bit like my family. We're a close-knit group and we talk to them and we share our worries" (volunteer).

There were opportunities to undertake training to do various health roles, and some of the courses were accredited. Although most volunteers were retired and did not want to apply new skills to employment, some had gained sufficient confidence to run sessions in group activities. Several spoke movingly of the transformative effects of volunteering on their lives:

> "Yes it's very rewarding and the social aspect as well. And also it's built up my confidence again. Because I had to pack up work and I think being at home, I did start to lose a lot of confidence, because I was always very confident when I was working ... and what have you. And then that confidence seemed to start ebbing, you know and I think this has brought me out again. Because when I first started, I was quite quiet ... but now I'm sort of my usual mouthy self, you know." (Volunteer)

The reciprocal nature of participation was also evidenced in interviews with service users attending project activities. Although not carrying out formal volunteering roles, many of the service users spoke of their active involvement in the project, assisting with the planning and organisation of activities, and offering informal support to other participants in the groups. Several were also involved in other types of volunteering activity on the estate, again motivated by the desire to give something back and/or the social benefits. Notwithstanding the broader strategic framework for community engagement on the estate, talking to volunteers and service users highlighted that becoming involved is ultimately a very personal journey. Overall, the case study provides further evidence of the positive impact of volunteering (Casiday et al, 2008) and highlights the reciprocal nature of engagement processes where community members have capacity to move within a spectrum of participation from formal to informal roles (South et al, 2012).

Embedded in the community

One of the strongest themes was the role of the volunteers in bridging the gap between the community and local services. This was a locality characterised by social and economic deprivation, yet the community was depicted as being tight-knit, with people "fiercely proud of their area". The project volunteers, who were described as "firmly rooted in [the estate] and their communities and their families and their networks", were therefore well placed to connect with other community members and give professionals a link into the neighbourhood.

This happened in a number of ways both formally through relationships built in the project, and informally outside as volunteers went about their daily lives on the estate.

The presence of the volunteers and their ability to make service users feel at ease was a key factor in facilitating residents' participation in the project activities. Helping tasks, such as welcoming people, making tea or running a raffle, were low-intensity, but it was these actions that ensured a comfortable and supportive environment that was appreciated by service users.

Lay designation – being a "normal person" – helped the volunteers relate to people accessing health services. One of the volunteers explained the value of peer support in encouraging service users to give up smoking:

> "I used to smoke ... and they tend to like support from ex-smokers. And from a normal person that can understand what they're going through day to day. And in fact they say, 'Oh it's been so many weeks' and 'I still', I said, 'I've been seven years and I still get sometimes, I still fancy a cigarette. But it goes ...'. We give an awful lot of emotional support more than anything else." (Volunteer)

Outside of the project, the volunteers were active in cascading health messages informally through their daily activities and social networks. Being well known and embedded within the community meant that residents were willing to speak with them and listen to what they had to say. Many local people just called into the project premises, and the volunteers, and also the project staff who lived on the estate, were often approached and asked for advice when going about the estate.

Health improvement activities could be promoted on the estate. A practitioner described how despite struggling to set up community-based smoking cessation services in other areas, what had made it succeed on the estate was having "someone from the community who knows the community, who has a passion for improving that community as well or working with that community".

Communication was not just in one direction. Like the sexual health project, involving volunteers meant that there was a point of connection through which community views could feed into planning and decision-making processes. In line with the original rationale of increased community involvement, volunteers in the community health committee brought their insights and shaped the development of project activities. Service users were asked their opinions, and suggestions for activities were taken forward in the project.

Identity and trust were recurring themes (South et al, 2011a). Volunteers, and also project staff who were local residents, were reported to be recognised and accepted in the community, although sometimes trust took time to build. There was perceived to be a natural resistance to those from outside the area and many residents were reportedly reluctant to seek professional advice: "Because a lot of people in authority don't look like they're living round here, and it's the same in a lot of neighbourhoods, there's like a real them and us I think" (staff).

The bridging role of volunteers was, therefore, a key mechanism to enable community members to access services, information or support. As one volunteer explained:

> "We can talk to them in their own language that they can understand, because we're just normal people. And I think they trust us because we are normal people. And they take on board what we say, whether sometimes we stumble and try and cover it up because we've made a big mistake somewhere, you know, but we're only human at the end of the day. And I think we get through to quite a few people, don't we? Because they trust us. I think it's trust." (Volunteer)

While lay designation was a key factor in community acceptance, it reportedly unsettled some professionals, who could "look down their noses" at the volunteers. One example of professional resistance can be seen in the failure to secure support for a leg ulcer group where people could join in social activities and have their leg dressed by a community nurse. This idea was rejected as the project building was decreed as a not sufficiently sterile environment. One individual reflected on the reluctance of professionals to let go:

> "People will talk the talk but when it actually comes to letting go or someone does something they're like 'Oooh', you know, they're straight away defensive and looking for the flaws rather than thinking 'Oh well that's great, that's people doing'. Because people are making choices daily about their health and ... we want people to be making the right choices, not forcing them." (Staff)

Sustainability – what is the price?

The neighbourhood health project demonstrated a high level of community participation, both in terms of intensity of activity and increasing community control, and this undoubtedly underpinned its success in reaching out to the wider community. Paradoxically the goal of handing over control to the community was threatened by over-reliance on a small group of volunteers. Volunteers demonstrated high levels of commitment to the project, but there was little turnover and new people were not being drawn in. Volunteers, many of whom were retired or had health issues, typically talked about their need to be available all the time because they "don't want to let anybody down" and sometimes "feeling pressured" and tired. The perception was that people were overstretched and this was a real threat to sustainability: "How are we going to survive, that is, because there's only sort of about four of us who volunteer, I mean, we can't stretch any further. You know, it's really tough" (volunteer).

Questions were raised about the appropriate level of responsibility for volunteers. There were challenges in being involved in democratic decision-making processes and putting in applications for funding. While forming a self-governing management group was seen as a laudable aim, professional support was required to underwrite this community-led action, for example, in writing funding applications. One volunteer explained that the thought of having to run the group completely by themselves was "quite daunting" because "there is so much red tape today".

Several of the people we interviewed questioned the extent to which the concept of handing over control was feasible or fair. One strategic lead talked about the responsibilities associated with the community committee in terms of an analogy with a local football team:

> "Actually, it's very few of the players that want to be the club secretary, to attend the disciplinary hearings, you know, to make the thing work, to apply for funding, they want to get on and do. And so why should it be a surprise that volunteers who you then try and turn into administrators and managers actually don't want to do that? They want to do the other stuff, you give them both roles, they get very tired." (External partner)

Interestingly, the issue of payment was raised as a potential means to reward the volunteer contribution. The volunteers could claim expenses, for example, for travel, but there was often a reluctance to claim and most just paid their own expenses from their own pockets. Some questioned the lack of financial compensation to people who in effect worked for free in the project, often putting in long hours. One service user, for example, commented that it was "a shame that they don't get anything for what they do" and a volunteer brought up the issue of rewards:

> "I mean, we go out for lunch, we've got to pay for it ourselves. But maybe they should say, 'Thank you for all the time you volunteer for us' and say, you know, take them out, give them a Christmas lunch. Yeah. It's not so much a reward, more like a thank you, you know what I mean? Yeah, all the good work that they've done over the year and that sort of thing." (Volunteer)

One major threat to sustainability was the expectation that project funding would come to an end as the regeneration programme scaled down and eventually closed. The logic that the community health committee would generate funding for activities was not completely flawed, as the committee had successfully applied for some monies. However, the scale of the task, to move to a self-funding, self-governing project, was regarded by many as a step too far. Interviewees were concerned about the impact of the end of regeneration funding and the competitive environment for bidding. One volunteer, for example, explained the challenge of juggling finances for Tai Chi classes to ensure that it became self-funding through subsidies, while the project paid for the hall rental. Furthermore, paid project staff were regarded as an essential component to provide the hands-on support to volunteers.

What can this model offer?

The neighbourhood health project provides strong evidence of the value of rooting health promotion activities within communities, particularly where those communities are disadvantaged. The approach was not about 'using' lay people to give professionals access to a community reportedly cautious about outside assistance, although undoubtedly the project did offer a vehicle for improving access to professionally directed interventions such as smoking cessation. Instead, the case study provides an example of how structures for genuine partnership-working between local services and the community can be built. Partner organisations – the council, the regeneration programme and the public health directorate in the Primary Care Trust – were signed up to the principles of citizen involvement and there was evidence that participation had genuinely heightened community influence.

Volunteers showed high levels of commitment; however, many of the volunteer activities in the project could be characterised as low-intensity, described as helping out. The case study shows that this type of informal activity was nonetheless critical in facilitating the involvement of local residents. The comfort factor should not be dismissed, as the bridging role of the volunteers, talking in the same language as the wider community, broke down barriers to accessing information and services. Notwithstanding the overt differences between the Community Health Educator model described in Chapter Eight and the neighbourhood health project, both case studies provide evidence to support the rationale for lay health workers as social and cultural connectors (American Association of Diabetes Educators, 2003; Rhodes et al, 2007). It is argued that such roles offer a mechanism to address health inequalities and improve connections between the state and society in line with the principles of both active and social citizenship (South et al, 2011a). A critical perspective needs to be maintained, as the services they are bridging between may be far from adequate.

Lay as opposed to professional designation, combined with identity and credibility within the local community, were all important factors. Here, the volunteer role spread beyond the boundaries of the project, and because volunteers were embedded within local social networks, they were able to take out messages. The conclusion is that placing these types of roles under heavy professional direction would be counterproductive. It is the bottom-up nature of the enterprise that delivers its success:

> "Because it's community-based, that's really the key to it. I mean sometimes certain communities especially respond very well to people from their own community, people they know, faces they trust often

and – and I guess that's really worked in [the estate] in my experience."
(Staff)

Despite the strengths of the community organising model, the case study also highlights dilemmas in seeking to build community capacity to deliver health promotion. The delivery of project activities was completely reliant on a small band of volunteers who admitted they were overstretched. There were threats to funding and evident need for some organisational support to underpin the functions of the community health committee. These findings suggest that the process of handing over control to communities needs to be adequately resourced and a broad base of volunteers needs to be built before the community can be expected to assume responsibility. As discussed further in Chapter Ten, citizen involvement should not be about the abandonment of statutory responsibilities.

Key points

- This case study of volunteering in a neighbourhood health project provides an example of citizen engagement in project planning and delivery.
- Volunteers demonstrated high levels of commitment to the project and to their community, but also gained personal benefits that reinforced their participation.
- As lay health workers who were living in the neighbourhood and trusted by residents, the volunteers were able to successfully bridge the gap between professional services and local people.
- The premise was that community participation would lead to sustainability as community members eventually took control, but the project was increasingly reliant on a small group of overstretched volunteers. The fairness and feasibility of the move to community-led management was questioned.
- The case study shows that genuine citizen involvement is achievable, and while it can deliver better relationships between services and communities in the short term, it needs to be accompanied by long-term investment to build community capacity.

TEN

Commissioning and delivery

This chapter discusses the key challenges in commissioning and implementing health improvement programmes that engage volunteers and members of the public in lay health worker roles. It builds on the previous chapters, in particular, the case studies and what can be learned from them about how to develop best practice. The effective engagement of lay people in improving the health of their communities needs a whole-system approach that is holistic in nature (Hunter et al, 2010). A whole-system approach makes it possible to see the interactions between different elements of the system and avoids reducing complex issues to component parts and thereby missing vital interconnections.

Since the People in Public Health study was undertaken, the public sector has experienced unprecedented cuts in funding, which have impacted on Primary Care Trusts, local authorities and the voluntary and community sector in major ways. In this policy context, there is an increasing emphasis on services being provided by the third and private sectors (Cabinet Office, 2011), and an acceleration of a trend to a mixed economy of welfare provision previously encouraged by the New Labour government (Ware and Todd, 2002; HM Treasury and Cabinet Office, 2007). The voluntary and community sector is seen to offer the independence, flexibility and specialist expertise that is often absent in the public sector and, more critically, to provide a bridge to some underrepresented groups (Bolton, no date; Billis and Glennerster, 1998). The recent NHS Future Forum report *Choice and competition. Delivering real choice*, which was concerned with strengthening marketisation levers, argued that 'there is a wealth of talent and untapped resource in our country's third sector which can benefit the NHS, so there is a good argument for greater commissioning from alternative providers of care where appropriate' (NHS Future Forum, 2011a, p 9). The size and diversity of the sector is considerable, for example, in 2002, it was estimated that there were more than half a million voluntary and community sector organisations in the UK (HM Treasury, 2002). Notwithstanding the significance of the third sector, it should be remembered that public services also support volunteering and involve large numbers of volunteers in public service provision.

A critical consideration, therefore, is what are the best delivery mechanisms for health improvement programmes engaging lay health workers: statutory, voluntary/community sector, social enterprise or private? The People in Public Health case studies were varied in terms of where delivery organisations were located and how services were commissioned. This chapter presents evidence and examples drawn from practice to argue that lay health worker programmes, wherever located, can only flourish, particularly in disadvantaged areas, if they are adequately funded and effectively managed.

The focus of the chapter is on the challenges that need to be addressed to ensure effective commissioning and implementation of lay health worker programmes, but it does not offer a prescription of how to engage volunteers. Programmes that are rigidly organised 'top down', like the original Expert Patient Programme, can be difficult to implement on the ground, especially when the agencies (in this case Primary Care Trusts) charged with their delivery have little or no experience of engaging volunteers (Kennedy et al, 2005a; Rogers et al, 2006). Flexibility is key; what works in one area will not necessarily work in another and there are no short cuts to careful thought and discussion with communities and other partners to determine what is needed in different contexts. Nevertheless, it is possible to learn from the experience of others, and to develop guidance on the issues that need consideration (see 'Engaging the public in delivering health improvement. Research briefing for practice', developed from the People in Public Health study [South et al, 2010a]). This chapter works through the different issues for public health practice, starting with commissioning.

Effective commissioning for health improvement and citizen involvement

Effective commissioning for health improvement needs to take a whole-system approach based on the five elements of the Ottawa Charter (World Health Organization, 1986), which was the first to summarise the foundations of health promotion and is still the bedrock of health promotion activity across the world. The five essential elements of health promotion are:

1. building healthy public policy;
2. creating supportive environments;
3. strengthening community action;
4. developing people's personal skills; and
5. reorienting health services.

A whole-system approach enables commissioners to commission 'solutions' not just services (Shircore, 2009) and recognises that a focus solely on individual behaviour change is not effective in improving health in the long term. Rather, what is needed is a commissioning approach that recognises the many factors that affect individual circumstances and choices. Shircore argues that commissioners should draw on those with health promotion and social marketing expertise to enable them to take a developmental approach to commissioning, starting with collaboration on a joint strategic needs assessment and followed by ongoing dialogue with all affected partners, including providers.

Clearly, if a whole-system approach to commissioning for health improvement is adopted, then deciding whether, where and how to commission for the involvement of lay people within health improvement programmes needs to be considered strategically rather than on a service-by-service basis. It needs to be part of an overall approach to commissioning that values community engagement, is grounded in community development principles and is developed in close collaboration with community organisations. Community development principles include recognition that people have skills as well as needs and have the right to participate in matters affecting them (Foot and Hopkins, 2010). Smithies and Webster (1998) represent how a whole-system approach to community development is needed with organisational, professional and community infrastructures in place to support community action on the ground (see Figure 10.1). As the Commissioning Support Programme (Commissioning Support Programme and Kindle, 2010, p 2) argue, it is for commissioners to ensure that community organisations are able to engage fully with the commissioning process:

> Engaging with community organisations in the design, delivery and evaluation of services through commissioning ... is an essential part of ensuring an effective and efficient suite of local services that respond to local needs. The challenge for commissioners is to ensure that those organisations feel able to engage fully with local commissioning processes and that their full potential is unleashed.

Figure 10.1: Essential elements of a community development strategy

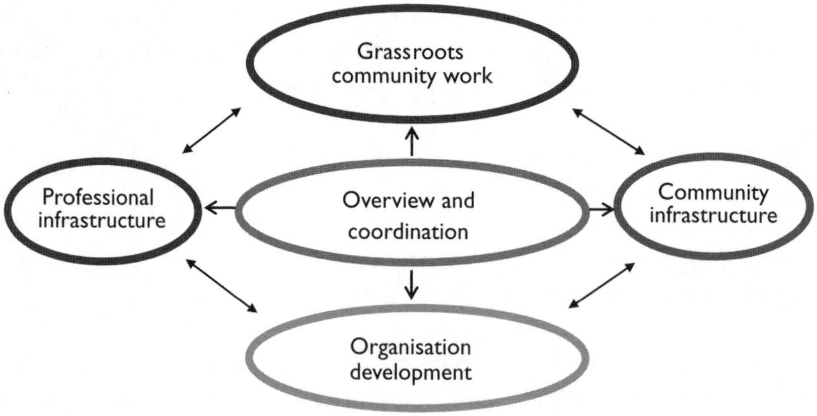

Source: Smithies and Webster (1998, p 238).

Box 10.1 presents an example from NHS Sheffield, where commissioning for community engagement has been built into their strategic approach within public health.

Box 10.1: Commissioning for community engagement in Sheffield

For many years, Sheffield has run an Introduction to Community Development and Health (ICDH) course, which seeks to empower people drawn from the more disadvantaged parts of the city to make their 'own informed choices, access services more appropriately and develop the skills and confidence to enable them to take advantage of opportunities which may become available'. More than 1000 people have completed the course and have gone on to become active in improving their own and their community's health in a variety of ways, including volunteering as a community health champion.

One example of a joined-up approach to community engagement is the diabetes work. Individuals with diabetes (or a close family member with diabetes) volunteer with Altogether Better Diabetes to support others to better self-manage their condition. They work closely with health trainers; many of whom were first graduates of the ICDH course, then community health champions and now work as paid health trainers. Both community health champions and health trainers are working with primary care as part of GP care pathways for diabetes. This joined-up approach has been developed by the Public Health Directorate in NHS Sheffield in partnership with primary care and is beginning to show very positive results in terms of better outcomes for people with diabetes.

Collaboration with the voluntary and community sector is central to the success of the ICDH course and community health champion and health trainer programmes in Sheffield, with NHS Sheffield commissioning community organisations in the most disadvantaged areas to deliver these on its behalf. Doing this in an integrated way, rather than commissioning each service separately, is building towards commissioning for community engagement as part and parcel of the mainstream.

Source: NHS Sheffield (no date).

The theme of commissioning was explored through the People in Public Health study in the expert hearings and the case studies (South et al, 2010b). At that time, the NHS was in the process of moving to World Class Commissioning (an organisational competency framework introduced by the New Labour government to improve the quality of commissioning health and care services) and commissioning within the health sector was still in its infancy (Department of Health, 2007). Not surprisingly, practice varied, with one participant at the expert hearings commenting that her Primary Care Trust operated with a medical model and had not been very good at commissioning the third sector in the past. Although there was a risk that the traditional patterns of funding would continue, she saw World Class Commissioning as an opportunity to enable more voluntary sector organisations and lay people to become providers, and to become involved in decisions about the prioritisation of investment.

In the People in Public Health case studies, some commissioners favoured a 'hands-off' approach, leaving the detail to the providers. While this recognises that the expertise around specific issues generally lies with providers, in reality, it usually means that the infrastructures needed to supported volunteering and community engagement, as outlined in Smithies and Webster's (1998) model, are not funded. This is one aspect of the tensions between professional and community control that was a theme running through the study. Another strong theme was related to health targets, where significant tensions were apparent between reporting on narrow targets determined by public health priorities and recognition of the wider social benefits of involving lay people. In the Walking for Health case study (see Chapter Six), for example, the change of focus towards tighter targets had profound implications for practice:

> "Nationally and locally it is the agenda, obesity, so I can understand why the focus has to be very target-driven. Obesity is now in provider services, so it's very much a matter of proving that the target that was given has been achieved. So anything else can't be catered to, so walks for mental health and social well-being can't really be catered to." (Staff)

Longevity of funding was also a key issue that came up time and again in the expert hearings and case study interviews. One community activist at the expert hearings described her frustration when it took 18 months to build the community support needed to get a project up and running to then find that the funding was gone. Citizen involvement takes time to get under way, as relationships and infrastructures have to be built. Continual uncertainty over funding is unsettling and demoralising for both staff and volunteers. A whole-system approach to commissioning implies ongoing support for community infrastructures that facilitate engagement.

New commissioning models

As organisations develop ways to involve citizens in controlling their own health and well-being through volunteering, they can be frustrated by existing systems of commissioning. This is because existing systems rely on cause-and-effect evidence, are geared to responding to specific clinical conditions rather than responding holistically to the needs and aspirations of individuals, assume delivery by technical experts, and rely for governance on corporate systems. There are emerging models that seek to provide a more inclusive approach to commissioning, one that opens the door to services rooted in communities. These might include a mix of service provision from professionals, unqualified staff and volunteers. Two examples of this, both the result of work funded by the Department of Health, are 'Thanks for the petunias' (Year of Care, 2011; see Box 10.2) and 'Tell us what the problem is and we'll try to help' (Gamsu, 2011). 'Tell us what the problem is and we'll try to help' captured and analysed the commissioning experience of five leading voluntary sector/social enterprise organisations in the North West of England. All of these organisations had services built around voluntary sector involvement and included the Lesbian and Gay Foundation, Self Help Services and Wirral Citizens Advice Bureau (CAB). Starting from the premise that the current commissioning environment, while not perfect, is susceptible to influence, a range of similar strategies for engaging with and influencing NHS commissioners were developed. Actions included:

- using volunteer and community experience to co-design solutions to 'wicked issues';
- capturing impact using accredited NHS information systems;
- proactively influencing upwards by building the capability of commissioners to understand the policy and evidence better; and
- contributing to local commissioning plans, rather than just responding to procurement opportunities.

Box 10.2: 'Thanks for the petunias'

'Thanks for the petunias' focuses on offering 'new, practical and cost effective ways to increase the opportunities for self management for people with LTCs [long-term conditions] by engaging with local non-traditional providers (e.g. charities, community organisations and social enterprises) to meet their needs' (Year of Care, 2011, p 5). It offers a model that seeks to provide pathways between medical and social models of health, making clear the pathway between self-care, minimal support, moderate support and high support.

The model proposed is one that fills in the pieces that have traditionally been missing from the commissioning jigsaw, which has traditionally placed the greatest emphasis on the relationship between the commissioner, the GP and individual service users. 'Thanks for the petunias' provides a more inclusive model, giving a more central role to non-traditional providers, who would employ health link workers, have strong local links to other non-traditional providers and provide a knowledge and information database to be used locally. This recognises the importance of connection and social engagement, which often has a voluntary component, either by the public or through connection with volunteers who are providing services. The commissioning model, which is based on a wide range of practical examples, seeks to address many of the deficits in the current system, notably, financial sustainability, more person-centred services, a strong focus on inequality, the need to increase social capital and capturing unmet need.

Source: Year of Care (2011).

Evidence from the People in Public Health study and elsewhere would support the view that where commissioning is undertaken in collaboration with community organisations, providers and users, and is part of a strategic approach, it is far more likely to be effective. Partnership work is demanding and time-consuming but essential to both a whole-system approach in public health and effective implementation (Hunter et al, 2010). The Department of Health endorses partnership-working as vital to the promotion and support of volunteering in health and social care (Department of Health, 2011b). Effective partnerships need to include the public and voluntary and community organisations on an equal basis, providing the support that community members may need to participate fully and ensuring their expenses are covered.

As Health and Wellbeing Boards are established as part of the changes to health and social care structures, and public health moves into local authorities, which are generally more experienced in working with disadvantaged communities than Primary Care Trusts, this offers opportunities for community engagement (Kuznetsova, 2012). Building stronger links between communities and services has the potential to radically alter the way public services are structured and run, through giving lay people a real say in programme planning as well as engaging them in delivery (for further discussion, see Chapter Twelve). Organisations commissioning or providing health services need to consider how they can systematically engage lay people. This includes how programmes are managed and how volunteers are recruited, trained and supported (see Box 10.3). These issues are considered in more detail in the rest of this chapter, after discussion of different service models.

Box 10.3: Questions commissioners need to consider

- How do services value the contribution of members of the public who are working to improve health in their communities?
- Do services develop and support people who can provide a bridge between services and communities?
- How well do services minimise barriers to engagement, recruitment and retention?
- Do people have good access to support in their roles?
- How do services ensure that people have opportunities to develop skills and knowledge?
- Do service targets reflect the wider benefits of citizen engagement in terms of addressing health inequalities and promoting social inclusion?

Source: South et al (2010a, p 5).

Service models

As described in Chapter Three, programmes involving lay health workers in delivery are diverse and have been adapted across a range of health issues, populations and settings. The People in Public Health scoping study mapped out a range of programme dimensions (South et al, forthcoming), which was later developed into a framework that set out the options available for those commissioning and developing local public health programmes (South et al, 2010a). This was intended to assist commissioners and managers in drawing up service specifications. Clarity about service models will help in building an evidence base, as lessons can be shared across programmes using similar approaches. The framework has four main programme dimensions, with key questions that need to be considered in designing local services (South et al, 2010a):

- **Intervention** – what is the programme trying to achieve?
- **Lay role** – what will members of the public do?
- **Service delivery and organisation** – how will professionals support this engagement?
- **Community** – what is the relationship with the community that the programme aims to engage?

Figure 10.2: Lay health worker programmes – four dimensions

Intervention	Lay role	Service dimensions	Relationship with community
What is the health focus? Who are the target populations? What are the programme goals? What are the intervention methods?	What is the primary role working with the target community? • Peer education • Peer support • Bridging – connecting services and communities • Community organising – mobilising community resources to address health issues Will the volunteers or lay workers work autonomously after training or require supervision by health professionals?	Who is the best delivery organisation? • NHS • Local authority • Voluntary sector • Social enterprise Training – will the emphasis be on preparation for delivery or on personal development and empowerment? Will there be any payment? • Volunteer model • Sessional payment • Employment model • Mixed	Will lay workers use their community knowledge and tap into existing social networks or will they be expected to build new networks? Is peer status important as part of the recruitment criteria? • Peer – matched to target population • Not matched to target population, but bringing general life experience • Embedded – known and working in own community

Source: South et al (2010a, p 3).

Effective leadership and management

The Department of Health concluded in their strategic vision for volunteering that: 'We need committed leaders and managers across sectors and across health, public health and social care who recognise that volunteering and wider social action are central to the provision of flexible and responsive services' (Department of Health, 2011b, p 19).

The People in Public Health study found evidence of some effective leadership within both commissioning and providers. Clearly, it is important for commissioners to provide leadership and to take a strategic, whole-system approach to commissioning for citizen involvement, as argued earlier. Managers within provider organisations also need to provide leadership, as do those engaged in research in this area, whether based in academic institutions or elsewhere. At the expert hearings and in interviews with managers and commissioners, participants stressed that leaders were needed who would seize the opportunities presented by organisational changes and new policy drivers to do things differently. Unfortunately, very often, when organisations are restructured, innovative policies are developed, but the people in power and organisational cultures remain largely the same. Effective leaders at whatever level challenge the status quo and are open to new ideas and agendas, but if there is little or no organisational support, then the innovation dies when that person moves on:

> "It has traditionally been reliant on the drive and perseverance of committed individuals. If you look at the breastfeeding issue, breastfeeding peer support groups, it's a committed midwife or a committed health visitor who has driven that forward. It hasn't come strategically from the top tier of the PCT [Primary Care Trust]."
> (Expert hearing 3)

Not only do managers need to provide leadership, but it is also vital to have effective management of programmes to improve health if they are to run smoothly. In their evaluation of the Expert Patient Programme, Kennedy et al (2005a, 2005b) found that, in general, managers in Primary Care Trusts did not have the time or skills to manage volunteer tutors effectively. There were many examples of effective, committed managers within the People in Public Health case study projects who displayed a wide range of competencies and skills, including some that were different from those needed to manage a paid workforce. Gaskin (2003) notes that in volunteer management, choice, flexibility and informality need to be retained; a point echoed by the Department of Health in its strategic vision for volunteering (Department of Health, 2011b), which stresses the need to reduce the bureaucratic barriers to volunteering while still managing risk effectively. It calls for volunteering procedures that are 'proportionate' to the role someone is undertaking (for further discussion of health policy on volunteering, see Chapter Two).

Volunteer management entails grappling with some thorny issues around role boundaries, risks and quality assurance. These need careful management through training, clear protocols and support mechanisms, as illustrated by Chapters Six and Seven. In addition, those managing programmes that engage members of the public in delivery need extensive people skills and experience of working with communities. They need an understanding of health improvement approaches and in-depth knowledge of the issues that are the focus of their programmes. All the above entail a wide range of high-level skills. As the Department of Health has recognised, engaging volunteers is not a cheap option and effective, properly resourced management infrastructures are vital (Department of Health, 2011b), a view echoed at one of the expert hearings:

> "The other issue about volunteers is that very often services see them as a cheap option. Actually, they shouldn't be a cheap option because you need a volunteer coordinator who's going to provide support for the volunteers and if you don't put in training, then you're not going to get anywhere anyway. So there are issues about costs that again statutory services don't always recognise." (Expert hearing 1)

Providing support for volunteers is essential if they are going to stay and develop their roles within public health programmes (Gaskin, 2003; Hawkins and Restall, 2006), as illustrated by the case studies presented in Chapters Six to Nine.

Working with professionals

The relationship between lay health worker and professional appears to be a crucial dimension to lay engagement and is highlighted in some of the key discussion papers (Eng et al, 1997; Dennis, 2003; Kennedy et al, 2008a), as well as being a major topic of debate at the expert hearings. Eng et al's (1997) notion of a continuum from natural helpers through to para-professionals integrated into a health service is useful. Many examples in English public health practice can be placed on that continuum, with some lay health workers trained and working independently and some working routinely alongside professionals. Table 10.1 provides a worked example of the continuum from assisting with a professional service to independent action. It would equally be possible to sketch this continuum in terms of increasing level of complexity/skill required in undertaking the task, for example, from simple information-giving, through to taking blood pressures, advice-giving and even counselling.

In each of the People in Public Health case studies, health professionals worked with lay health workers, and, in some cases, were employed within the projects. Some participants reported that health professionals saw lay health workers as lacking relevant knowledge and skills:

> "I think some of the professionals boo hoo us." (Volunteer)

Table 10.1: A continuum of volunteering using the example of a health promotion group session

Increasing independence	
	Service user who helps make the refreshments/puts the chairs out.
	Service user who brings the milk and stays behind to lock up.
	Volunteer user who promotes the session and welcomes newcomers.
	Volunteer who books speaker/facilitator and room and organises the session.
	Volunteer who leads the session.
	Volunteer who does above and liaises with professionals about the session.
	Volunteer who does above and liaises with professionals not just about the session, but also about broader direction/policy, attending meetings, giving updates and so on.
	Volunteer who does all of the above plus takes forward issues raised by the group and lobbies for change.

> "I think they [lay workers] need credibility, I think they need that, I think a lot of health care professionals see themselves as the professionals and they know best." (Staff)

Failing to gain acceptance from professionals could be problematic. For example, in the Walking for Health case study (Chapter Six), it had proved difficult to get GP referrals, although there were positive examples where GPs supported the scheme and allowed walks to meet outside the surgery. Some GPs were reportedly sceptical about the scheme:

> "The GPs were scared because again people making a claim and how can they refer people onto something that they weren't directly in control of, you know. And yeah, I think their biggest issue was someone would trip over and fall and make a claim. I found the health care professionals quite hard to get around. The community sector, the voluntary sector, you know, most people were open to the idea and said 'Yeah that's logical let's work on it'." (Staff)

The professional–lay relationship was not a major focus of the study; however, it appeared that the initial scepticism of health professionals often moved to acceptance and support after experiencing working with volunteers, showing that acceptability is fluid and something that can be built up over time.

The way that health services operate, indeed, their organisational culture, can be a major barrier to citizen involvement (South et al, 2011c). In both the expert hearings and case studies, respondents talked about the 'top–down' nature of the NHS being a barrier, with local health organisations very focused on medical matters that could be at odds with local communities. Some health professionals clearly felt threatened and did not understand what lay people can offer.

Arguably, it is the nature of professions to define an area of knowledge and expertise and to resist what they see as the intrusion of anyone not qualified to work in that area. So, for programmes engaging volunteers to experience resistance from professionals, whether dieticians, health visitors, teachers or even, at times, community development workers, is perhaps not surprising. It is also important to acknowledge that professionals have genuine and, at times, justifiable concerns regarding risk and quality. During this period of public sector cuts, there are additional fears about less-qualified staff or volunteers replacing professionals (for further discussion, see Chapter Eleven). There are, however, many professionals who support the engagement of lay health workers, particularly when they have experienced how well this can work to support them in their work with communities. Box 10.4 provides an example of where paid and volunteer peer supporters were an integral part of a health service.

Box 10.4: Breastfeeding support – an integrated approach

One of the People in Public Health case studies was of a breastfeeding peer support programme. Volunteers were recruited via breastfeeding support groups and trained to provide support to new mothers. Some progressed to paid peer support worker posts and one went on to train as a midwife. At the time of the interviews, there was a core staff of part-time paid peer supporters who worked between 16 and 25 hours a week, arranged flexibly to fit in with childcare and family commitments. Paid peer support worker roles involved:

*   providing information about the benefits of breastfeeding in the antenatal period, on a one-to-one basis, in the home or at various groups;
*   visiting the postnatal wards at the local maternity unit to support new mothers;
*   one-to-one home visits in the days following birth and as required in the postnatal period; and
*   working closely with local Children's Centres and voluntary breastfeeding support groups and referring parents to local support groups.

There was volunteer input, as volunteers helped run breastfeeding support groups and encouraged pregnant women to attend these to find out about breastfeeding. In addition, the programme provided a 24-hour telephone line that had some volunteer involvement. Overall, both paid and volunteer lay health workers complemented rather than replaced the role of midwives and health visitors. There were clear role boundaries and training was part of managing risk as well as preparing for roles. Case study participants, including service users, identified benefits in the involvement of peer supporters who were perceived as:

*   'normalising' rather than 'medicalising' breastfeeding;
*   being more available and having more time to spend with mothers; and

- being more acceptable to mothers and able to empathise, and, in some cases, speaking their first language.

A number of challenges were also identified, including:

- determining what were appropriate roles for volunteers and paid peer supporters, differentiating these from professional roles, and ensuring that volunteers did not go beyond their role;
- ensuring volunteers received adequate training and support;
- covering expenses – especially for childcare; and
- overcoming professional scepticism and ensuring referrals were appropriate.

Source: South et al (2010b).

Recruitment and retention

Identification, recruitment and selection of lay health workers are all important processes that need consideration in developing lay health worker programmes. There are differences between programmes where identification and recruitment is professionally led and tends to be more formal (Britten et al, 2006), and ones where it is community-led and more open. A further issue, highlighted in some of the international literature, is the significance of using recruitment methods where the community of interest assists in identifying 'natural helpers' within the community and recommending them as lay health workers (Eng and Smith, 1995; McQuiston and Uribe, 2001). Recruitment strategies can evolve depending on community response and often diverge even within a common model (Jackson and Parks, 1997).

In public health practice in England, the ways in which lay health workers are identified and recruited vary considerably, as borne out in the People in Public Health expert hearings and case studies. There was a spectrum in the case studies from largely professionally led recruitment with specific selection criteria in the breastfeeding peer support project, to open-ended, community-led recruitment in the neighbourhood-based and Community Health Educator projects (Chapters Eight and Nine).

Using inclusive and flexible approaches to recruitment is important, as it allows a range of people, including those from disadvantaged communities, to step into public health activity. People with local knowledge of their communities, with what one speaker in the expert hearings described as "street intellect", have much to offer. Having life experience, commitment and insight into the community were more important qualities than prior knowledge or formal qualifications. One programme represented at the expert hearings did not apply any selection criteria, and had a policy of recruiting people for what they could offer, not what they lacked. In some instances, this meant that individuals were recruited who had significant problems of their own:

> "We had a community member whose children were on the at-risk register, so all the health professionals we've ever worked with have been lovely to us but they said "How can you have somebody going out teaching somebody about healthy living when they can't even look after their own kid?" ... She never worked with kids and what she did do was a lot of first aid work for us and healthy cooking. So it's employing people for what they can do and not for an absence. Her kids are not off the at-risk register, but you can understand how controversial that is, it's a big challenge for us." (Expert hearing 2)

In community-based programmes, recruitment may happen in an informal way largely by word of mouth, as illustrated by the case studies in Chapters Six to Nine. It becomes necessary to formalise recruitment processes in order to manage risk when volunteer roles involve more responsibility, but this can become a barrier to recruitment. The Expert Patient Programme, for example, struggled with recruitment in the early years of the programme, and had little reach into disadvantaged groups (Rogers et al, 2006). For those disadvantaged communities, the normal organisational channels of recruitment are unlikely to work, in particular, advertising through the internet and written applications. One of the expert witnesses described how she had recruited successfully by providing a staged approach whereby people could initially come to an informal open session about health, then get a certificate of attendance for participating in a series of informal workshops, before deciding whether to commit to the full training programme.

Recruitment by word of mouth, using local networks and contacts, is an effective strategy, as demonstrated by the case studies (Chapters Six to Nine). Community groups, such as the local church, and community-based activities, like festivals, and other types of informal settings can be used. The breastfeeding peer support programme, for example, recruited many peer supporters through breastfeeding support groups in the community. Service users also helped with recruitment by passing on information and recommendations to family and friends. In most case studies, there were examples of service users making the transition to being volunteers or paid lay health workers (for discussion of the volunteer journey, see Chapter Five).

The case study projects also used more formal advertising methods of recruitment, such as project websites, posters in community health centres, local publications (particularly newspapers) and leafleting households. The organisation hosting the sexual health outreach project had their volunteers wear T-shirts with 'I am a[n organisation] volunteer speak to me about volunteering' written on them. Recruitment was not always easy, for example, despite their high visibility in the community, the neighbourhood health project was struggling to gain new volunteers (see Chapter Nine).

Barriers to recruitment were not explored in depth in the case studies, but it was noted in the expert hearings that bureaucratic procedures were often in conflict with organisational aspirations to engage the community:

> "through CRB [Criminal Records Bureau] checks, they had to go through quite a tough interview process, they had to sign a document saying they would do certain things during the year. And that was at odds with the limited responsibility a lot of people expect from a voluntary role." (Expert hearing 3)

Literacy was identified as a barrier, but, at the same time, there were examples of how this could be overcome through inclusive recruitment processes and support as required.

Managing recruitment is one of the key roles of managers and demands some different skills and approaches to recruiting to paid jobs. For example, the Community Health Educator programme had various volunteer roles on offer to enable people to start with something relatively undemanding. Those that were interested and able could then progress on to more demanding roles (see Chapter Eight).

Building confidence, for example, through providing opportunities to progress, is key to retention. In addition, it is important to provide relevant, appropriate, accessible training and ongoing support, so that lay health workers always have somewhere or someone to turn to if they need help. The People in Public Health study found access to 'light-touch' support was a critical factor in ensuring effective delivery and a positive experience for volunteers. Payment and expenses as a form of support is explored later in the chapter. If lay health workers feel appreciated and support systems are in place, then retention is likely to follow.

Competencies, skills and training

Programme managers need to be clear what competencies and skills are required for lay health worker roles and ensure that adequate training has been provided to enable lay health workers to undertake their role safely and effectively, even where these roles are relatively low-intensity or informal. Volunteer roles can demand a very high level of skill and sophistication (see Chapters Six to Nine), and are by no means at the low level ascribed to them in the Public Health Skills and Career Framework (Public Health Resource Unit and Skills for Health, 2008). Training in the case study projects was of varying depth and length depending on the service, and served a number of purposes as well as preparing people for the role they would undertake. Personal development was a strong theme, reflecting Shiner's (1999) distinction between training for peer delivery and training for peer development. Access to training could prepare people for a working role more generally, providing a stepping stone into employment. Training enables people to meet other volunteers and project staff (Hainsworth and Barlow, 2003) and, particularly where it runs over a number of weeks, helps build relationships.

Accrediting training can prove important not just to provide evidence of competence, but also to build self-esteem. Accreditation through organisations like the Open College Network can be at various levels and is done through portfolios that do not necessarily demand high levels of literacy, while, at the same time, providing a way of ensuring quality and that learners gain credit for what they have achieved (see Box 10.5).

The content of training needs not just to cover the health issue(s) to be addressed or the role that the lay health worker will play, it is also an opportunity to explore the project's values and approach, introduce new ideas, and encourage participants to question. In discussing the development of a college credit certificate for community health workers, Love et al (2004) argue that having a core curriculum enhances employment mobility and professional acceptance, and also develops community health workers' critical thinking through an understanding of the social determinants of health. This approach is also reflected in the Leeds Community Health Educator course (Box 10.5).

Box 10.5: Leeds Community Health Educator course

All Community Health Educators do a 14-day course (10am–2.30pm) for one day per week before getting involved in work in the community. The course is described in the project literature as 'experiential and excitingly innovative where individual definitions of health are explored in the context of the community'. Course modules explore who learners feel has power over them and how this can impact on their health. The students can elect the health topics that have validity and meaning in their everyday lives. Ideas and experiences are shared and there are no textbooks. The course is designed to raise consciousness and increase confidence levels, health and employability, and uses informal, arts-based and interactive methods. On the course, students learn:

- to be an effective health promoter, making people aware of the potential risks to their health and how to improve their health;
- how to organise and run group activities;
- about the health issues in their areas and how they can be improved;
- how to examine issues about inclusion and how race, religion and culture influence people's attitudes; and
- how to find out what resources, services and networks are available.

The course is accredited by the Open College Network and students can achieve up to 15 credits at level two. Most Community Health Educators go on to do further training and get involved in a wide variety of volunteer and paid work.

Source: Healthy Living Network Leeds (2010).

All training needs to cover governance and risk-management issues and to ensure that lay health workers understand the boundaries of their role and when to seek help. The structure of the project needs to be clear as to how lay health workers will access support and other resources. Programmes dealing with sensitive issues like HIV/AIDS need to pay particular attention to these issues (Kelly, 2004), as was clearly evidenced in the sexual health outreach case study (see Chapter Seven). The level of skill and competence displayed by the volunteers in this case study was particularly high and the need for them to be clear about the limits of their role was paramount.

Training can be a means of filtering out individuals not ready for a volunteer role, or to determine what sort of role they could undertake. As the case studies illustrate (Chapters Six to Nine), having a range of training opportunities opens up opportunities for people to follow their interests, as well as to develop in the role and ensure that they are up to date. Several of the case studies had experienced volunteers who went on to train others, alongside paid staff trainers. Trainers need a wide range of skills and competencies geared to training people who may have had a poor experience of education or not taken part in any formal learning for some time. Training groups of people whose self-esteem and confidence is low can be challenging, but also very rewarding. The level of skill and stamina required should not be underestimated and ensuring training is adequately resourced is a crucial part of programme management.

Training is one of the key ways in which risk is managed and good governance is assured (for an example, see Chapter Seven). Risk falls into three areas: potential risk to the volunteers themselves; potential risk to the public or service users; and potential risk to the organisation and/or its paid staff. Training can be a key strategy to ensure that lay health workers develop the competencies required for the role (Berrios, 2002), and to build acceptance from the professional community (Love et al, 2004). The staff in the case studies were very aware of risk-management issues and of the need for a balanced approach. This is discussed in depth in the context of the sexual health outreach project, where staff were proactive in ensuring that risk was anticipated and managed effectively (Chapter Seven), and in the Walking for Health scheme (Chapter Six), where the volunteer role was independent of services.

Payment and expenses

Payment and expenses is a complex area and the People in Public Health study revealed a variety of different models. The question of how rewards and remuneration should be handled remains contested territory. The focus of this book is on volunteering and lay health worker programmes that use sessional payments to support engagement, rather than those programmes that incorporate lay health workers within employment structures. Health trainer services, for example, usually employ health trainers on Agenda for Change band 3 (which started at £15,860 in 2011). There is often an assumption, reflected in UK policy, that there is a clear distinction between volunteering and paid work, for example, the recent *Strategic vision for volunteering* (Department of Health, 2011b, p 9) defines volunteering as: 'Activity undertaken freely that involves spending time, unpaid, doing something that aims to benefit the environment or individuals or groups other (or in addition to) close relatives'.

In contrast, literature on lay health workers shows a variety of models (Jackson and Parks, 1997; Taylor et al, 2001; Lehmann and Sanders, 2007). Furthermore, the relationship between low-paid work and volunteering has been questioned (Baines and Hardill, 2008). Various approaches to rewards and remuneration were debated at the expert hearings, and the five case studies represented different payment methods, which allowed the research team to explore views on the models available. The neighbourhood health (Chapter Nine) and sexual health outreach (Chapter Seven) case studies were volunteer-only programmes, as was Walking for Health (Chapter Six), although there had been a history of sessional payment for some walk leaders. The breastfeeding programme had both paid and unpaid roles, with peer support workers receiving a wage of around £14,000 pro rata, and the Community Health Educators (Chapter Eight) were paid on a sessional basis. The range of models for remuneration has been summarised in Table 10.2. This section explores some of the advantages and disadvantages to the different approaches to payment and expenses.

Payment has been found to have a number of advantages for public health programmes. Remuneration, and also employment, of lay health workers was associated with greater reliability and accountability:

Table 10.2: Models of remuneration for lay health worker programmes

Independence

Independent community activism – no financial support from services, for example, self-help groups, community campaigns.

Volunteering – with volunteer claiming for out-of-pocket expenses. May cover aspects like travel, substance, childcare, phone usage.

Volunteering with agreed allocation to cover out-of-pocket expenses and any additional occurred expenses, for example, £10 a session for walk leaders.

Financial incentives for attending training or recruiting participants, for example, shopping vouchers.

Sessional payment based on type and number of activities attended. May or may not include additional expenses claimed separately.

Sessional payment based on hourly rate, akin to temporary working arrangements.

Employment with organisation, with variable hours depending on duties.

Regular employment with organisation.

Employment models

"One of the reasons that [project name] works is because it's paid support and when you pay people they're accountable for what they do. So I could say to a volunteer "I've got a mum that needs seeing on Monday, are you free?" and she might say "I might be but I'm not sure". If it's a paid worker I know she's available because she's at work from 9 'til whatever." (Expert hearing 1)

However, another expert witness speaker cautioned that payment could alter the dynamics between the lay health worker and their community:

"Once people are in a paid job you are changing that dynamic. We learned some difficult lessons as a result of employing someone from the Gypsy and Traveller community without giving enough thought to the tensions she would experience. It put her in a completely different situation with the people that she lived with. We must look at those implications." (Expert hearing 3)

Pay can give credibility to a role, provide a sense of worth to the lay health worker and demonstrate appreciation for their contribution. One Community Health Educator explained: "The rate I got paid was fantastic … it made you feel even more wanted and worthy". Research from other lay health worker programmes suggests that payment can help with retention (Leaman et al, 1997; Taylor et al, 2001; Lehmann and Sanders, 2007). Remuneration can make it possible for people from disadvantaged groups to contribute, something that came through strongly in the Community Health Educators case study (Chapter Eight), and, furthermore, can help with employability. Yet there was no evidence that it undermined altruistic motivations:

"I find that I have other things to do that mean really I don't want to see it as a wage, I don't want to see it as doing so many sessions a week so that I get paid so much money. So I'm not looking at it as a sort of a paid job, it's just something extra to do besides the voluntary work." (Community Health Educator)

There are disadvantages associated with pay. It can be seen to conflict with the volunteer ethos, which would help explain why some lay health workers in the case studies would refuse expense refunds (see later). In the expert hearings, the fear was expressed that pay would make it more difficult to get programmes mainstreamed because of the expense. There could be tensions where volunteer and paid lay roles coexisted, but, conversely, where lay health workers were paid the same rate, this raises the issue of equity as individuals' capabilities and responsibilities differed (see Chapter Eight). In contrast, the Walking for Health scheme had previously chosen to pay specific volunteers because financial support was considered necessary to secure their involvement (see Chapter Six):

"We paid some volunteers, but it was very specific ones, it was people who were unemployed who had to go out of their way to come. It wasn't a case of paying volunteer expenses, it was more if people were employed in whatever capacity, then they got nothing, but if you are unemployed and you really need this money to get to it, you know, that sort of thing." (Staff)

In both the expert hearings and in those case studies that involved people below retirement age, there was a call for clarity regarding conflicts between benefits and payments/incentives for lay people:

"What needs to be in place is a system to support these people during that process, and not just people on incapacity benefit, but all people so they can start by volunteering as a way back into employment, and that they need to be supported in having an additional allowance rather than losing any of their benefits. Because there needs to be incentives to encourage people to volunteer and not barriers, which seems to be what's there at present." (Expert hearing 3)

Managing pay and expenses is an issue for programme management. Remuneration is particularly important to support participation for those on benefits because they are surviving on a low income. Consequently, the risk of losing benefits is magnified because that income is precious:

"It's not a vast amount of money and it shouldn't affect the benefits. If it affects the benefits then their husbands will get a bit wary, "If it's going to affect our benefits then what will happen when you stop doing it" and that kind of thing, so leave it, it's not worth it." (Staff)

The People in Public Health study found that although staff planned to cover expenses and to avoid any financial burden on lay people, this was complicated to achieve. Hidden expenses still occurred and remained difficult to claim, for example, obtaining receipts with the use of pre-paid mobile phones. In the breastfeeding project, childcare was a prominent personal expense, and one individual explained how they covered her volunteering by her husband coming home early from work, but as he was on hourly pay, that this was costing the family money. Some volunteers were reluctant to claim expenses, even in the neighbourhood health project, where volunteers put in long hours and were likely to be on low incomes or benefits (see Chapter Nine).

While payment can be a factor supporting participation, where projects were based on volunteering (see Chapters Six, Seven and Nine), absence of remuneration did not mean that people felt unrewarded, as social rewards, such as companionship, enjoyment, sense of purpose and personal satisfaction, were viewed very positively. Service users tended to view volunteer status as signalling a commitment to the community, but, at the same time, in both the Walking for Health scheme and the neighbourhood health project, there was some discussion around the extent of responsibilities and the lack of remuneration:

> "As a volunteer walk leader there is only so much free time you can give for nothing and I think [name] has found that it's encroached more and more on his personal time which he has found. Well, it's fine to a point but then you get to a point where you think, well, you'd like to take it further, but to take it that much further you need that financial reward to say 'Yes, this is a job effectively'." (Service user)

It will be clear from the earlier discussion that there are no 'right' or 'wrong' answers about payment. It helps if the principles are determined strategically at the district if not national level, but individual services will need to decide what is the best model depending on factors such as the financial position of those they want to recruit, the nature of the roles to be undertaken and the level of training and responsibility involved. Careful consideration needs to be given to issues of equity as people take on different levels of responsibility, and the issue of benefits and expenses needs to be actively managed, not left to individuals. Finally, while payment is an important and potentially thorny issue, in general, people do not get involved for the money (see Chapter Five). Therefore, making volunteering enjoyable and appreciating people's contributions remain just as, if not more, important than payment.

Conclusion

This chapter has discussed the main issues that need to be addressed if engaging the public in programme delivery is to be effective. If involving volunteers and other lay health workers is seen as an 'add-on', which requires little or no support and is expected to be cost-free, then it will fail. A level of investment and an infrastructure that actively addresses barriers to involvement are both required (South et al, 2010a). The approach should not be about imposing top-heavy organisational structures on grassroots activity. It should be about developing systems that are flexible and supportive and ultimately enable members of the public to play a role in health improvement. It is also about challenging old ways of working and looking for new models based on true collaboration between commissioners, organisations, practitioners and the communities they serve. Chapter Twelve expands on ideas for a new way of working, after having 'debunked' some of the myths about citizen involvement and volunteering in Chapter Eleven.

Key points

- This chapter has discussed what public services need to do to support the involvement of members of the public in programme delivery in an effective and sustainable way. Key issues around commissioning, management and implementation have been explored.
- A whole-system approach is required for commissioning, one that recognises the potential for partnerships between active citizens and professional services and provides ongoing support for community infrastructures that facilitate engagement.
- Professional leadership, management, support and training are critical to ensure recruitment and retention of volunteers and effective delivery of lay health worker programmes.
- Some of the issues within practice, such as payment, are complex and require active management, as well as critical reflection. There is no standard model for implementation or any recommended approach; each programme needs to consider its role with lay health workers in relation to the setting and community needs.

ELEVEN

Dispelling the myths

Throughout this book, evidence has been presented of ways in which lay people are improving community health and what needs to be in place to enable them to do this effectively. This chapter takes a step back to consider whether citizen involvement is necessarily a 'good thing' and to explore and challenge some of the counter-arguments about lay health workers and active citizenship in health. These counter-arguments can be broadly categorised into four:

1. 'It's a diversion, as only addressing structural inequalities will improve health and address inequalities.'
2. 'Involving lay people is too risky – professionals are needed.'
3. 'If it's work, people should be paid for it – involving lay people threatens jobs.'
4. 'It might be nice to do, but where's the evidence?'

These four arguments have been called myths because the authors believe that while there are important issues and concerns underpinning some of them, they are all fundamentally flawed. By contrast to these four myths, which are all sceptical of citizen involvement, there is a fifth, neoliberal argument that is dominant in UK politics, which is that citizen involvement is good because it makes it possible to cut services and 'shrink the state' as people take more responsibility for themselves. While the reality of a smaller public sector is all too real, the appeal that community activism will spontaneously grow once the Big Society replaces big government is another myth (see Hunter, 2011). This chapter critiques all five myths and sets out some alternative arguments supporting citizen involvement in the context of current public health challenges. These arguments are developed further in the final chapter, which explores some new ideas that are gaining currency and sets out a manifesto for change.

Citizen involvement is a diversion from addressing structural inequalities

Health is socially determined, and macroeconomic conditions are powerful forces that shape population health (World Health Organization, 2008a). Recent publications such as The Marmot Review (2010a) and *The spirit level* (Wilkinson and Pickett, 2009) have demonstrated that the social gradient of health is damaging to all sections of society. Put more simply, more unequal societies have worse health outcomes for all.

While health inequalities are regarded as unjust because they are seen as amenable to change, there seems little consensus on precisely what strategies are most effective. New Labour public health policy demonstrated tensions between policy oriented to improving living and working conditions through multi-sectoral action (Department of Health, 2003) and policy oriented to maintaining a focus on individual behaviour change and choice (McKee and Raine, 2005; Scott-Samuel and Springett, 2007). Earlier chapters have presented evidence and examples that position lay health workers as part of a strategic approach to addressing health inequalities because of their ability to reach into and work with communities facing barriers to achieving good health. In some quarters, this strategy is seen as a diversion from addressing the 'real' issue of changing macroeconomic conditions, and, moreover, it is regarded as ideologically suspect, linked to a neoliberal discourse on individual responsibility and a smaller state. Taylor et al (2011, p 6), for example, suggest that those on the Left regard the Big Society drive to devolve local services and strengthen communities as 'putting a sticking plaster over the wound caused by macro-structural inequalities in power and resources'. This section challenges the myth that citizen involvement is necessarily a 'sticking plaster', and argues for a more nuanced understanding of the relationship between the state and society.

In a typology of actions to tackle the social determinants of health, Whitehead (2007) argues that interventions based on strengthening individuals in disadvantaged communities are of limited value because they only treat the symptoms and not the underlying causes of inequalities. The underpinning logic is that societal causes should be addressed by societal-level solutions, achieved through state action. Expecting individuals and families to take responsibility for addressing health inequalities is seen as 'victim-blaming' and, ultimately, unfair and futile. While macro-level solutions are undoubtedly required, these solutions are much more likely to come about if citizens are engaged, and through this, become more aware of the reality of inequalities and, therefore, see the need for system change (Wallerstein, 1992). As Chapter Four discusses, the link between equity and participation is central to health promotion policy and practice.

The welfare state is intended to equalise life chances, yet not only is there a failure to achieve this mission (as the post-war trends in health inequalities in the UK show), but also services can unintentionally reinforce the existing power gradient. Disadvantaged communities need welfare services (benefits, housing, social care etc) more than other groups in order to mitigate the effects of market forces, yet power imbalances in society mean that public goods are distributed unequally. The Marmot Review (2010a) demonstrates that there is a social gradient in the characteristics and conditions of healthy communities. The inverse care law, first described by the socialist GP Tudor Hart, applies here: those most in need are likely to have the least good access to services (Hart, 1971). Watt (2002) argues that co-morbidity in disadvantaged areas means that families often have multiple, severe and complex health and social problems. This can lead to social exclusion of some groups, for example, the Travelling community, who find it difficult to access even basic-level provision. Lay health workers have been a proven resource that can improve the reach of services and reduce barriers to access for marginalised communities, and can therefore be an important strategy for addressing health inequalities (see, eg, Lam et al, 2003; Andrews et al, 2004; Perez-Escamilla et al, 2008; Open Society Foundations, 2011). In each of the case studies presented in Chapters Six to Nine, bridging was identified as a key function, even in low-intensity interventions, enabling communities to make connections to the resources needed for health.

Citizen involvement is not only about improving access, it is also about redressing inequalities in power. State services very often create dependent and passive citizens because of the way they are structured and operate (North and Peckham, 2001). This passivity can be detrimental to the health and well-being of those citizens, as well as unsustainable. The lay voice can be excluded, and groups like mental health service users risk stigmatisation (Beresford, 2001; Opinion Leader Research, 2001). Incorporating a lay element in service provision can help humanise services and therefore break down barriers for less-advantaged groups (see Chapters Seven and Nine). The 'comfort factor' should not be underestimated, as research with service users shows (Flax and Earp, 1999; Faulkner, 2005). Involvement of lay people, as service users or members of the public, can also transform the way services are organised, with huge benefits for users and staff alike. Neuberger (2008) argues that volunteering is important in health and social care as it helps reorient services and indirectly promotes cultural change. Lay health worker programmes can therefore be seen as a means to alleviate power imbalances and improve citizen control.

A final justification for citizen involvement is the imperative for action to prevent the immediate effects of health inequalities. Critical health issues faced by communities require focused action in the short term, as well as long-term macroeconomic solutions. The different levels of intervention are not mutually exclusive. Lay health workers can offer an effective means of addressing social determinants, such as social support, where major inequalities exist, while making a crucial difference to individuals at risk or experiencing poor health (see Chapter Four). Figure 11.1, for example, shows the inequalities in social support, as presented in The Marmot Review (2010a, p 136).

It is interesting that while the health trainer initiative has been critiqued for its focus on individual behaviour change (Trayers and Lawlor, 2007), clients drawn from less-advantaged communities consistently rate the service very highly and see the relationship with their health trainer as making a real difference to their confidence to achieve health goals (Kime et al, 2008; White et al, 2010a; White and Kinsella, 2011). Health trainers do not solve the structural inequalities that fundamentally determine people's health, but they do support people to gain confidence and start taking control of their lives where they can. As Tones and Tilford (2001) argue, this individual empowerment is a necessary prerequisite to community empowerment and social action.

Framing volunteer or lay-led services as essentially a distraction from tackling the structural determinants of health is therefore posing a false dichotomy. Both are needed to address inequalities and both are essential to build a new public

Figure 11.1: Percentage of those lacking social support, by deprivation of residential area, 2005

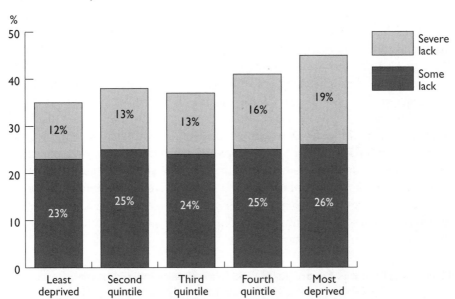

Source: Health Survey for England (2005). Copyright © 2012. Reused with the permission of The Health and Social Care Information Centre. All rights reserved.

health movement, as proposed in Chapter Twelve. An example of this dual approach can be found with the Haamla service in Leeds, which provides peer support and education to black and minority ethnic women, including asylum seekers and refugees (Kinsella et al, 2009). The cultural support provided by both paid lay health workers and volunteers is valued by the women as making the essential difference to their immediate experiences and their engagement with other services. Haamla is both an ethical and pragmatic solution to the immediate challenge of better birth outcomes for this vulnerable group of women, but one that needs to be part of wider strategies to address health inequalities and improve access to maternity services.

Involving volunteers and lay health workers is a credible response to health inequalities, but this response should be within a citizenship framework that emphasises rights as well as responsibilities, in line with recent international policy statements (World Health Organization, 2011; World Health Organization Regional Office for Europe, 2012). Volunteer involvement can be framed as representing both active citizenship and social citizenship, as it is about promoting greater equity in health and improving connections between the state and society (South et al, 2011a). There is an undoubted risk that those who have least are expected to 'plug the gap' where services are inaccessible or provision is under-resourced. Public health is essentially a political activity (Bambra et al, 2005) and the authors would concur with the need for continued advocacy, ideally from disadvantaged communities themselves, to improve the living and working conditions for all and to transform the way services are organised (Carlisle, 2000).

In summary, strategies are needed at all levels of society, including those at an individual and community level. Creating and developing healthy and sustainable places and communities is one of six policy objectives emerging from The Marmot Review (2010a). Citizen involvement is about addressing social determinants, whether that is through strategies for democratic renewal or enabling people to take small steps to good health (World Health Organization, 2011). Figure 11.2 shows how strategies to increase citizen power can fit with macro-structural solutions, whereas low levels of citizen involvement are likely to reinforce the status quo. Empowerment is about people having more control over their lives and their health and this is associated with positive health outcomes (Wallerstein, 2006). This is not just about feeling better – empowered communities can begin to access resources to which they are entitled and advocate for changes in the distribution of resources, ultimately challenging the socio-economic conditions that lead to health inequalities.

Figure 11.2: Power and strategies for addressing health inequalities

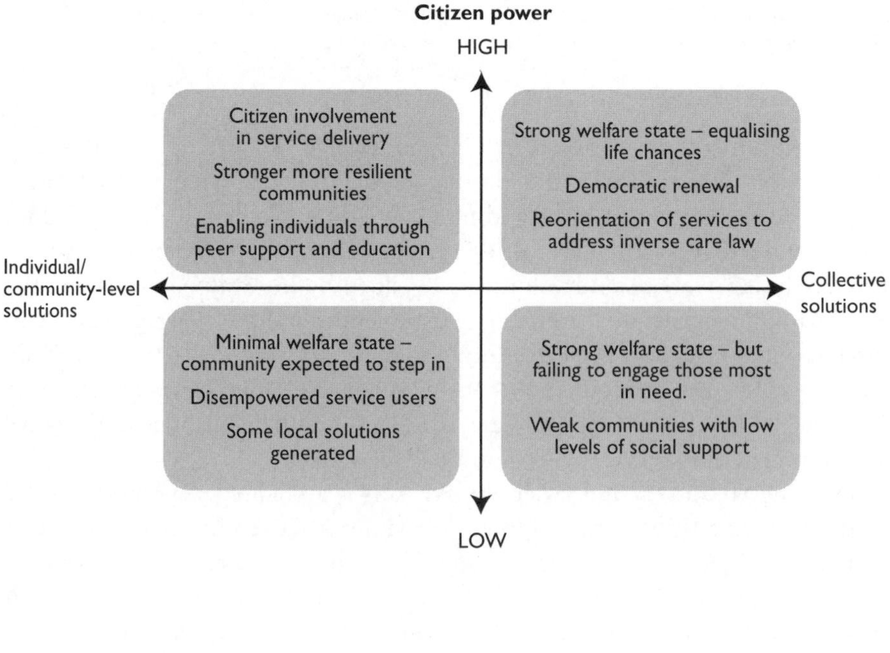

This work needs a professional

Many lay people working to improve health are doing so alongside health and social care professionals, or have people referred to their scheme by a professional. Moreover, those managing public health interventions that involve lay people will almost certainly be engaged at some level in partnership work with professionals.

This section discusses the nature of professionalism and the linked concept of 'medicalisation' in order to provide a context for the issues that can arise around the lay–professional interface. Some of the criticisms levelled at professions, particularly the medical profession, are briefly reviewed, but there is also recognition of some of the challenges that professionals have faced in recent years. The conclusion is that the health and social care professions will need to continue to adapt as new models of working that are more inclusive of lay people come to the fore.

Professionalism has both positive and negative sides. Professionalism can be defined as expert and specialised knowledge in a field. Foucault (1977, p 27) has argued that 'power and knowledge directly imply one another' and with the 'old' professions, such as law and medicine, it is clear that claiming a monopoly on an area of knowledge has been used to gain both economic and social power. The medical profession has grown and sustained its power in part through the medicalisation of more and more areas of life from pregnancy, birth and death to ageing and the way we live. A recent editorial in the *British Medical Journal* (Godlee, 2010, p c4766) argues that doctors, through developing new diagnostic categories like 'pre-hypertension', 'pre-osteoporosis' and 'sarcopenia' (age-related loss of muscle), are not only opening up potentially profitable new markets for drug companies, but are in danger of 'transform[ing] most of the world's adult population into patients'. Arguably, the medicalisation of large parts of everyday existence, such as eating or being physically active, provides a role for professionals where maybe only a limited one is warranted. This is not to contend that understanding the early signs of, for example, diabetes or the long-term effects of obesity are not important; the question is whether these are best addressed using a medical or social model of health.

The power that the medical profession continues to exert over many areas of society has long been criticised by sociologists, alternative therapists, the women's health movement and others (see, eg, Illich, 1975). Other clinical professions such as nursing and midwifery have often been in conflict with the medical profession over role boundaries and so it is perhaps unsurprising that when lay people start in engage in health work, this can give rise to suspicion and resistance. Research on breastfeeding peer support, for example, points to potential conflicts and boundary issues arising between peer supporters and health professionals (Dykes, 2005), with some health professionals actively gatekeeping and being territorial with volunteers (Curtis et al, 2007). Professional resistance, where it occurs, is not limited to the involvement of volunteers, but is often experienced when 'skill mix' is introduced into practice and the professional groups affected fear that their role is being undermined by the involvement of less-qualified staff (Prentice, 2011). In the past, initial resistance has often evaporated when the benefits of sharing tasks and complementary roles became apparent. What Neuberger (2008, p 19) describes as the public sector 'aversion' to using volunteers can emerge from a lack of understanding of how volunteers can be integrated into health and social care services.

Acceptance of lay health workers should not be equated with devaluing the professional contribution. As well as defending areas of expertise against those deemed unqualified to practice, health professionals also have positive values and standards, which include a duty of care, confidentiality and putting client interests ahead of their own. Nursing, for example, is based on these values, plus equality, justice, utility, solidarity and humility (Rognstad et al, 2004), and the doctors' code of ethics, based on the Hippocratic oath, is still highly valued. Clearly, in times of need, everyone wants the assurance that they are being treated by someone qualified to a high standard and who has been rigorously assessed. Rather, the debate is about whether lifestyle is an area where clinical expertise is needed. For example, when does it need to be a dietician who advises about healthy eating and when can a lay person do this?

In recent years, positive aspects of professionalism, such as putting the interests of the client first, cooperation with other professions in the best interest of those clients and growing practice through reflection, have faced challenges from the growth of managerialism and, arguably, this has added to the defensiveness sometimes emanating from professionals. Managerialism is the belief that organisations have more similarities than differences, and, thus, that the performance of all organisations can be optimised by the application of generic management skills and theory. To a practitioner of managerialism, there is little difference in the skills required to run a college, an advertising agency, an oil rig or a volunteer programme in public health. Experience and skills pertinent to an organisation's core business are considered secondary and so decisions are made not based on professional expertise, and certainly not based on the views of the community served, but based on managerial prerogatives. This trend reflects neoliberal ideology and can be observed in relation to all professions; for example, in education, less and less value has been placed on the professional judgement of teachers and how they operate in the classroom is increasingly determined by others (Davies, 2003).

Similarly, nursing as a profession is facing huge challenges through managerialism, which is replacing the values that underpinned nursing and the welfare state with those of the private sector. It is argued that an emphasis on performance, targets and quality control is undermining care for patients and changing the very psyche of nurses as practitioners (Ball, 2007; Bosley and Dale, 2008). Nursing tasks are increasingly reduced and separated into individual components and 'health technicians' with limited roles are being employed to replace a nurse who (ideally) would take a holistic approach and provide continuity of care (Shields and Watson, 2007). This is not to argue that managers and management are not important. A recent Kings Fund report, which reviewed management and leadership in the NHS, concluded that: 'the NHS will be able to rise to the financial and quality challenges it faces only if the contribution of managers is recognised and valued' (The King's Fund, 2011, p vi). It is the model of management characterised by managerialism that is undermining health professions. This becomes the context into which lay health workers, both paid and volunteers, are being introduced, which goes some way towards explaining why these roles may be resisted by professionals.

The attack on professionalism is part of a wider attack on the welfare state, which those on the Right of the political spectrum blame for having created a 'culture of incivility, irresponsibility, family breakdown and disorder' (Phillips, 2007). The critique of professionalism advanced in this book comes from an alternative perspective that recognises the way in which doctors, medical institutions and public health have traditionally functioned as agents of social control (Conrad, 1992). Understanding what may lie behind professional resistance to lay engagement not only helps to develop strategies to form productive partnerships, but can also inform thinking about where programmes involving lay workers, such as health trainers, are best located. This issue is explored by Kennedy et al (2005b) in relation to the Expert Patient Programme, where the introduction of a new workforce of volunteer tutors was seen to bridge the gap between informal care and formal provision. The authors discuss some of the dilemmas arising from volunteer trainers becoming part of a professional (NHS) workforce; an issue that has also arisen in the Health Trainer Programme in England and in community health worker programmes across the globe (Witmer et al, 1995; Eng et al, 1997; Jackson and Parks, 1997; Levenson and Gillam, 1998). Understandably, for those who see volunteering or taking a low-paid lay role as a stepping stone to qualifications and better-paid work, gaining recognition for what they do is important and being seen as a 'professional' is generally viewed as of higher status than being 'lay'. Conversely, if programmes engaging lay people become too much a part of the public sector, lay health workers run the risk of being simply 'another pair of hands' working under professional control (Walt, 1990).

Moving away from a professional monopoly in public health inevitably entails greater acceptance of the lay contribution. As is demonstrated in Chapters Six to Nine, there are some things that lay people can do better than professionals and vice versa, and successful programmes draw on the strengths of both. The case study of breastfeeding peer support in Chapter Ten provides an example of where professionals and lay people are working successfully together. Challenges to the existing paradigm of Western health provision are now coming from some surprising sources. *Turning the world upside down*, a book written by Nigel Crisp, who was Chief Executive of the National Health Service and Permanent Secretary of the Department of Health until 2007, considers the dominant historical trend of Western scientific medicine as a movement towards greater professional competence, scientific discovery, commercial innovation and massive spending (Crisp, 2010). On the basis of his review of what works in poorer countries, he suggests an alternative paradigm where greater professional competence is achieved through patients and communities empowering and working with professionals and replacing measures of input spending by measures of social and economic value. The paradigm shift that Crisp proposes has many similarities to the core themes of this book. As a society, there is a need for a rebalancing of power in relation to everyday matters, like food choices, away from professional control.

This not only moves towards the 'fully engaged scenario' that Wanless (2002, 2004) argues is so critical for better health outcomes, but will provide the basis for true co-production in public health, as is explored in Chapter Twelve.

Volunteering threatens jobs

It is undoubtedly the case that some on the Right of the political spectrum see citizen involvement as a way of getting people to do jobs voluntarily that have previously been paid, underpinned by a neoliberal stance that seeks the reduction of the welfare state. The perceived threat of job substitution can be an obstacle to acceptance of volunteer roles (Neuberger, 2008), and this section provides a counter-argument by examining the more progressive view of volunteering emerging from the trade union movement. These debates, however, need to be seen in the light of the current economic situation, with the retrenchment of public services. The authors fundamentally oppose the replacement of paid staff by volunteers and support the position of workers and trade unions who are challenging the government policies that are leading to such substitution. Inevitably, volunteering is not always perceived positively by people who work in the public and voluntary sector during times of change, when services are being cut, reorganised or outsourced. The authors do not support the development of unpaid internships and work placements that last months and rarely lead to paid jobs, or proposals for those on benefit to be 'forced' to volunteer or lose their benefits, and would agree with those who see all these examples as exploitation (Helm and Asthana, 2010; Volunteering England, 2011).

Recognising that governments and employers may well seek to substitute paid jobs with volunteers does not mean that volunteering is necessarily a bad thing. The trade union movement has increasingly taken a more sophisticated view of volunteering. This is best described in a charter agreed between the Trades Union Congress (TUC) and Volunteering England in 2009 (Volunteering England and TUC, 2009). In this charter, there is a shared statement recognising that 'volunteering plays an essential role in the economic and social fabric of the UK' and is helping to 'build social capital and community cohesion and playing an important role in the delivery of key public services' (Volunteering England and TUC, 2009, p 1). Volunteering is recognised as being beneficial to volunteers themselves in terms of improved health and well-being and providing opportunities 'to acquire skills and knowledge that can enhance career development or employment prospects' (Volunteering England and TUC, 2009, p 1). The charter affirms the shared values between voluntary action and trade unionism, notably, mutuality and reciprocity, that can lead to positive changes in the workplace and the community and sets out some key principles to underpin good relations in the workplace (see Box 11.1).

Box 11.1: Volunteering – the trade union view

- All volunteering is undertaken by choice.
- While volunteers should not normally receive or expect financial reward for their activities, they should receive reasonable out-of-pocket expenses.
- The involvement of volunteers should complement and supplement the work of paid staff, and should not be used to displace paid staff or undercut their pay and conditions of service.
- The added value of volunteers should be highlighted as part of commissioning or grant-making, but their involvement should not be used to reduce contract costs.
- Effective structures should be put in place to support and develop volunteers and the activities they undertake, and these should be fully considered and costed when services are planned and developed.
- Volunteers and paid staff should be provided with opportunities to contribute to the development of volunteering policies and procedures.
- Volunteers, like paid staff, should be able to carry out their duties in safe, secure and healthy environments that are free from harassment, intimidation, bullying, violence and discrimination.
- All paid workers and volunteers should have access to appropriate training and development.
- There should be recognised machinery for the resolution of any problems between organisations and volunteers or between paid staff and volunteers.

Source: Adapted from Volunteering England and TUC (2009).

The charter's considered approach to establishing common cause between these two sectors is at odds with the view of trade unions as being the first to leap unthinkingly to challenge unpaid work. However, the charter should not be surprising, as the trade union movement has much in common with the values of voluntarism. First, it is based on the voluntary participation of its membership. When the charter was launched, Brendan Barber, the TUC General Secretary, noted that there are 200,000 union representatives in the UK, making the trade union movement one of the biggest volunteering organisations in the UK (TUC, 2009). It is also one that expects its volunteers to be involved in the whole continuum of volunteering, from practical activity, through to individual advocacy and wider political engagement. This reflects the very roots of trade unionism and its values of solidarity and mutualism (Hobsbawm, 1984).

Second, in addition to volunteers providing the bulk of trade union infrastructure, trade unions often support and promote many other forms of voluntary activity that impact on health and well-being. The TUC has a well-resourced infrastructure that includes key platforms such as 'Unionlearn',[1] which acts as a gateway and resource for the training of Union Learning Champions and other voluntary roles. The learning champion approach has many similarities with the health champion model, as described in Chapters Three and Ten. Health and safety representatives offer another example of voluntary roles. Again, the TUC provides a comprehensive package of support and training that includes advice about how to interpret statistics on workplace health. The TUC is clear that many of the gains that have been made in workplace safety arose from the voluntary activity of trade union representatives over the last 100 years.

Difficulties undoubtedly exist where lay people are engaged in voluntary activity that is very similar to the work others are doing for payment, and where volunteers want and need paid work. A Volunteering England publication on volunteers across the NHS (Hawkins and Restall, 2006) is clear that volunteers should add value and not be a substitute for paid staff. Chapter Four rehearses some of the key arguments for the distinctive value of lay health workers. These are difficult times to be advocating for more citizen involvement, but, as is argued in Chapter Twelve, there is scope to look at different and more effective ways of organising public health services. This presents challenges in terms of what is considered paid and unpaid work, and these boundary issues are particularly pertinent where communities face high levels of unemployment. Baines and Hardill (2008), reporting on a study of volunteering in a disadvantaged community, highlight the paradox that volunteering can be a positive choice for individuals but, at the same time, an adaption to labour market failure. These issues are equally complex in developing a lay workforce in public health and need working through in specific programmes. Ultimately, there needs to be wider debate about whether the boundaries between paid and unpaid can be viewed in a somewhat different way as part of challenging existing power structures and building a more egalitarian and less acquisitive society. As discussed in Chapter Ten, consideration should be given to appropriate levels of training and support and volunteer roles should be matched to levels of responsibility and also given fair rewards. These issues need to be carefully managed, but are not in themselves reasons for not supporting citizen engagement.

Lay engagement is not evidence-based

Public health in England appears to be in the grip of a grand obsession with evidence, which colours many of the debates about practical strategies to improve health and reduce inequalities. The drive to justify public health interventions on the sole criteria of robust evidence (using a hierarchy that places randomised controlled trials at the top) is combined with a commissioning culture narrowly focused on specific health problems, rather than improvements in the environments in which people live and work. All this creates a climate where community engagement approaches are forever on the 'back foot', struggling to prove worth, and in the current competitive world of cost savings, only what is considered the most methodologically sound evidence is valued.

This challenge is one that has its roots in wider debates about what is an appropriate evidence base for public health and how that can be built (Green and Tones, 1999; Kelly et al, 2002; Rychetnik et al, 2002). For example, Smith and Petticrew (2010), in an article subtitled 'Time to see the wood as well as the trees', are highly critical of current public health evaluation, arguing that, too often, macro-level interventions, like urban regeneration, are still evaluated using micro measures such as individual behaviour change. A further challenge for those wishing to develop an evidence base is the developmental nature of participatory approaches (Springett, 2001; Barr, 2003); the result being many 'practice stories' that are not easily generalisable (Burton, 2009).

Despite the strong theoretical rationale, and the wealth of evidence on good practice, there is often a sense that lay health worker programmes can never measure up to a quasi-clinical public health intervention, where the distance between cause and effect is short and individual-level change is measured in quantifiable terms. It is this myth of citizen involvement as nice but essentially fluffy, and certainly not based on evidence, that this section challenges. The arguments are twofold: first, to argue for wider acceptance of the current evidence base; and, second, to begin to construct a more fitting evidence framework for these approaches.

The National Institute for Health and Clinical Excellence (NICE) reviewed evidence on community engagement drawn from research and from expert opinion, and the guidance produced in 2008 recommends recruiting agents of change in local communities 'to plan, design and deliver health promotion activities and to help address the wider social determinants of health' (National Institute for Health and Clinical Excellence, 2008, p 28). As described in Chapter Four, there is already a strong evidence base for the effectiveness of community health worker programmes and peer-based interventions across different health issues. A rapid review undertaken for the Altogether Better programme synthesised evidence from a total of 19 reviews, including 14 systematic reviews (see Table 11.1). Evidence of positive effect was identified across a range of health outcomes (South et al, 2010c):

- increased knowledge and awareness of health issues;
- increased uptake of preventive measures such as immunisation;
- positive behaviour changes, particularly when working with disadvantaged, low-income or minority ethnic communities, for example, increased physical activity levels;
- improved disease management where programmes work with people with long-term conditions;
- more appropriate use of health care services, including reducing barriers to access and decreasing hospital admissions; and
- positive impact of volunteering on volunteer health, including better mental health.

There were inevitably knowledge gaps, such as evidence about wider impact on social networks, and inconclusive results, such as the effectiveness of lay-led self-care programmes for people with long-term conditions (Foster et al, 2007). Some of the wider impact of lay health worker programmes in communities may be difficult to capture, but assumptions should not be made about lack of

Table 11.1: Selected systematic reviews on lay health worker/peer-based interventions

Publication	No of studies included	Population and settings	Individual-level outcomes reported	Community-level outcomes reported	Cost–benefit reported
Bailey et al (2005) 'A systematic review of mammography educational interventions for low-income women'	24 8 on peer educators	Low-income or black, minority ethnic (BME) women	✓	✗	✗
Brownstein et al (2007) 'Effectiveness of community health workers in the care of people with hypertension'	14	Primary focus BME populations in US (most commonly African-Americans including four studies on African-American men)	✓	✗	✗
Corluka et al (2009) 'Are vaccination programmes delivered by lay health workers cost-effective? A systematic review'	3	Two studies on child immunisation One on older people	✓	✗	✓
Fleury et al (2009) 'The role of lay health advisors in cardiovascular risk reduction: a review'	20	Most studies related to vulnerable and underserved populations in US	✓	✓	✗
Lewin et al (2010) 'Lay health workers in primary and community health care for maternal and child health and management of infectious diseases' (Cochrane Review; update of Lewin et al, 2005)	82 21 from original review	International review Two thirds of included studies from high-income countries	✓	✗	✗
Norris et al (2006) 'Effectiveness of community health workers in the care of persons with diabetes'	18	BME populations in 16 of the 18 studies	✓	✗	✗

(continued)

Table 11.1: Selected systematic reviews on lay health worker/peer-based interventions (*continued*)

Publication	No of studies included	Population and settings	Individual-level outcomes reported	Community-level outcomes reported	Cost–benefit reported
Perez-Escamilla et al (2008) 'Impact of peer nutrition education on dietary behaviors and health outcomes among Latinos: a systematic literature review'	22	Latino population in US	✓	✗	✓
Rhodes et al (2007) 'Lay health advisor interventions among Hispanics/Latinos: a qualitative systematic review'	37	Hispanic/Latino communities in US	✓	✗	✗

Source: South et al (2010c).

effectiveness, as absence of evidence with social interventions is not the same as absence of effect (Petticrew, 2003).

Much of the available evidence originates from the US, where there is not only a more established tradition of lay health workers, but also a history of social experimentation with many large-scale intervention trials where changes are measured longitudinally, for example, the Expanded Food and Nutrition Education Programme (see Perez-Escamilla et al, 2008). Transferability of this evidence needs consideration, as the UK welfare state, including its public health system, is very differently structured. On the other hand, most of the US evidence is drawn from programmes working with low-income, minority ethnic or otherwise disadvantaged communities and therefore has relevance to addressing health inequalities in other contexts.

Overall, it is possible to conclude, based on review evidence, that lay health worker roles are an effective mechanism to promote health (for further discussion, see Chapter Four). There is a need to disseminate the existing evidence base and to debate its relevance in different contexts and with different communities, so that it becomes part of the planning process and is not used as a justification for limited short-term funding. There are good examples of where a comprehensive evidence base is being slowly assembled, for example, the Cardiovascular Health Awareness Program in Canada (see Chapter Three), and it should be possible to extrapolate from these demonstration projects to UK practice. Furthermore, there is room for commissioning models that balance scientific evidence alongside other types of evidence, such as community knowledge (Rada et al, 1999).

It is perhaps surprising given this evidence base that community-led approaches in the UK still feel the 'burden of proof'. There are a number of reasons for this, some of which go to the heart of the politics of public health. The array of terminology, and sometimes poor description of interventions in published research, makes it difficult to identify similar approaches and synthesise evidence (Lewin et al, 2005; National Institute for Health and Clinical Excellence, 2008). It is particularly frustrating when commonplace terms used in international contexts, like community health worker, are not used at all in UK practice, which seems to have its own lexicon of roles (South et al, 2010b). There is a danger of being overly insular and failing to draw on the learning from lay health worker programmes in the developed and developing world, where there is much grounded experience (see Chapter Three). A further problem is that funding for evaluative research in the UK has a biomedical bias and is rarely focused on macro-level approaches and wider public health impacts (Whitehead, 2010). Finally, the politics of evaluation mean that there is an institutional blindness to community-led interventions that tends to ignore or devalue lay knowledge. For example, individual narratives of the impact of participation are dismissed as anecdotal evidence and self-reporting is never regarded as being as robust as physiological tests.

Dispelling the myth of lack of evidence around citizen involvement is, therefore, much more than a dissemination challenge. It is also about tackling the paradigm that views public health evidence through a narrow prism, based on a traditional hierarchy of evidence. If the wider impacts of involving citizens are to be captured, there needs to be a better understanding of the nature of health programmes that seek to work in partnership with communities. As Chapters Six to Nine show, even where lay health workers deliver simple interventions, their work cannot be reduced to a set of neatly defined tasks. Active citizens are likely to be resources in their communities and act independently outside the boundaries of the intervention through their social networks, and the wider impacts can ripple through communities. Therefore, evaluation approaches need to start from a holistic view of health and be capable of capturing health and social impacts at community and individual levels over time (Nutbeam, 1998). There is value in using participatory research methods that can give voice to disadvantaged groups (Feuerstein, 1986; Moewaka Barnes, 2000; Minkler, 2004). Given the challenges of assessing the cost-effectiveness of community engagement, Mason et al (2008) recommend involving communities in research to help capture the full impacts, which currently tend to be missed.

A final point of debate is how lay health worker roles are seen: as an intervention or as an essential part of the health system? In evaluative studies, roles are usually framed as part of the intervention and therefore subject to testing around effectiveness. But what if lay health workers were viewed as part of a mixed economy of health, taking a rightful place in service delivery with other professional workers? Evidence would then need to focus on how effective lay workers were at reaching different groups, how well they supported and engaged people, and if they improved access to health services. If subjected to the same scrutiny, many mainstream health care services would not score well using these criteria. The Marmot Review (2010a) is evidence enough that our current welfare system has proved inadequate to deal with the challenge of health inequalities. The point being that the current burden of proof is partly to do with the way that the question 'Does it work?' is asked.

Volunteering and the Big Society – the view from the Right

These are ideologically confusing times, with much of the rhetoric on the Left and Right of the political spectrum being superficially the same. The government, espousing the Big Society, talks about 'empowering communities', 'opening up public services' and 'promoting social action' (Coote, 2010), all phrases that could equally be from left-wing publications that seek to challenge existing power bases. This section examines what some of the key think tanks on the Right of the political spectrum are saying about volunteering, and argues that it is vital to look beneath the words in order to understand the real ideological base of their ideas and whose interests they serve. Some of the think tanks maintain support for a traditional free market approach, while others seek influence across all political parties and, as the Social Market Foundation (Social Market Foundation, no date) states, 'marry markets with social justice' and take a 'pro-market rather than free-market approach'. This section looks at four of the major think tanks:

- ResPublica;
- the Social Market Foundation;
- the Institute for Economic Affairs; and
- the Policy Exchange.

ResPublica came to prominence through the work of its founding director Philip Blond and his book *Red Tory* (2010). The work of ResPublica underpinned much of the thinking of David Cameron's Big Society and both ResPublica and the Social Market Foundation have been particularly influential with both the New Labour and Conservative parties in recent times. *Red Tory* was an attempt to reconnect conservative thinking with a particular view of the past that claims that it was the Conservatives (or Tories) who were the original advocates for the poor and champions of society (Blond, 2010). According to ResPublica:

> The Big Society is about individuals and communities solving their own problems. Through mutual and reciprocal engagement people can make their own decisions about what is best for them and their communities and take an increased sense of responsibility for their lives. The Big Society is about building on the huge strengths, energies and skills that are already put to use throughout Britain. (Wilson et al, 2011, p 5)

In 2011, ResPublica published *Civic limits*, a report that sought to contribute to a 'grounded debate around how to get more people involved in civic life' (Wilson et al, 2011, p 3). According to ResPublica's analysis, there is a small 'civic core' of the population who undertake the majority of volunteering activity, quoting that 30% of the UK adult population contributing about 90% of all volunteer hours. It suggests that 'people belonging to this "core" are more likely to be well-educated and middle class than the population as a whole' (Wilson et al, 2011, p 3). *Civic limits* calls on the government to have aspirational targets to double the level of volunteering among adults, and, furthermore, takes an inclusive view of what volunteering actually is, recognising the relationship between individuals contributing and wanting to engage more in local decision-making. ResPublica is clear that volunteering and civic engagement will require government intervention and funding to increase the size of the 'civic core' through improving capability and reshaping the way in which services are commissioned and through policies created to build participation and engagement from the beginning.

The Social Market Foundation seeks to 'marry markets and social justice. It neither sees the market as a necessary evil nor as an end in itself but as a means to improve people's lives' (Social Market Foundation, no date, p 2). Like ResPublica, it has contributed to the debate on citizenship and shares a view that the role of government is not to avoid this agenda, but to 'unlock that massive potential and find new ways of harnessing the power of people to improve their own lives and those of their neighbours' (Bradley, 2007, p 40). This position was put forward in a polemical Foresight pamphlet that also promotes the idea that all local services could do more and do it better if they have more voluntary support:

> How much better for patients, practitioners and the health service if the voluntary groups which support the victims of chronic and debilitating conditions were not almost entirely made up of the patients themselves and their relatives? (Bradley, 2007, p 42)

Much of the discussion on the value of volunteers and the potential to promote more active citizenship chimes with arguments for greater citizen involvement in public health. What is missing from this discourse, however, is recognition that to engage patients, citizens and communities requires resources from the state to be effective. As Chapter Ten argues, unleashing people's potential requires a supportive infrastructure and good volunteer management (Gaskin, 2003).

The more traditional view from the Right focuses less on the role of civil society and more on the role of markets. The Institute of Economic Affairs (as influential with Margaret Thatcher as ResPublica was briefly with David Cameron) assertively promotes 'the intellectual case for a free economy, low taxes, freedom in education, health and welfare and lower levels of regulation' (Institute of Economic Affairs, 2010). Reflecting neoliberal ideology, the Institute sees markets as the best mechanism to address social and economic problems. In 2007, the Institute published 'Rescuing social capital from social democracy', which argued that 'government attempts to undertake "cultural planning" to create social capital are subject to exactly the same problems that lead economic and industrial planning to fail' (Institute of Economic Affairs, 2010). According to the Institute, for democratic systems to work, governments must be limited to coordinating core political functions, while markets will generate attributes such as trust and non-discrimination.

In general terms, the more libertarian the think tank, the less they have to say about the role of government with regard to citizenship and volunteering. This is because they do not think there is one. The focus of the Policy Exchange is on encouraging corporate social responsibility. Publications like *Building bridges: philanthropy strengthening communities* (Davies and Mitchell, 2008), with its introduction by Lord Eddie George, the former governor of the Bank of England, speak directly to the market itself, not to government. It proposes a recalibration of the private sector's moral compass and encourages an increase in philanthropy in terms of money and time.

Underpinning the words of the Policy Exchange is the view that choice in the market is the only driver for quality and value, individual responsibility is the mechanism for a good society and government is a barrier to individual freedom and success. ResPublica and the Social Market Foundation may not go so far, but still see the market as a potential power for good and the need to rein back on state power. These perspectives are somewhat contrary to mainstream public health, where the powerful negative impact of economic conditions on people's health has long been recognised and the need for coordinated action on the social determinants of health is advocated (Acheson, 1998; Wilkinson and Pickett, 2009; The Marmot Review, 2010b). Many in public health would see an urgent need to place limits on the activities of the financial sector and big business, as these continue to increase inequality with consequent harmful effects on health (Navarro, 2007; Stuckler et al, 2011). The state is a potential power for good, and support for a comprehensive welfare state is not incompatible with advocating for reform of public services to make them more inclusive and allow citizens more control.

Volunteering can offer a means to enable people to access services to which they are entitled and to enhance capabilities (South et al, 2011a) in line with the principles of social citizenship (Taylor-Goodby, 2009). The ideological position advanced in the book is thus in opposition to the right-wing ideology that underpins current government thinking, despite the congruency of much of the language used. Public health needs to reclaim this language in order to fashion a different approach that both seeks to defend the public sector and to reshape it. The welfare state is a vital part of this, but it needs to change to be more inclusive of people and communities. While the current policy context poses a genuine threat to living and working conditions, this should not obscure arguments for redefining the relationship between citizens and services. Chapter Twelve sketches what a public health system that fully engages its citizens might look like, and explores alternative ideas that might inform the creation of a society in which citizens are active in improving their health.

Key points

- This chapter has argued that the key objections to the involvement of lay people in public health activity are all flawed.
- Citizen involvement does not equate to saying that there are individual solutions to structural problems. It need not undermine professionals or replace paid jobs.
- Rather, there are good justifications, combined with a growing evidence base, that support citizen engagement as a way of addressing public health issues, redesigning services and giving people more control over their health.
- Rebalancing power in public health entails a critique of traditional ways of thinking.

Note

[1] See: http://www.unionlearn.org.uk/

TWELVE

Future directions

Introduction

If there is to be success in addressing the major health challenges of today, in tackling the social gradient of health and in promoting well-being in all sectors of the population, then public health needs to be done differently. The current public health system, the way the workforce is organised and the downstream focus on lifestyle interventions is evidently not up to the task in hand. Debate about public health capacity continues to focus almost exclusively on the capabilities and resources of professionals, rather than recognising the capacity of citizens and communities to make a significant contribution. Despite all the aspirational policy statements on citizen empowerment (Secretary of State for Communities and Local Government, 2008; Cabinet Office, 2010), and the importance of a fully engaged society (Wanless, 2004), the lay contribution is still not harnessed in any systematic or mainstreamed way. Knowledge about how to involve people has not been translated into the creation of an infrastructure to sustain that involvement in order to bring about long-term improvements in health. Yet the potential benefits that would result from 'putting the public back into public health' (Heller et al, 2003, p 62) would be enormous. This final chapter revisits the major themes of the book, bringing in some fresh perspectives that shift thinking on lay engagement. The chapter ends with a manifesto for change based on the value of active citizenship for public health.

The focus of this book has been the involvement of members of the public (lay people) in the delivery of public health programmes, one of the ways communities can play a larger part in public health efforts (see Figure 1.1 in Chapter One). The book has looked at why, how and with what support people can move from being passive consumers of services to active citizens who make a valued contribution to health improvement. The major themes for policy and practice explored in the book are topical, not least because of the current fiscal crisis and the threats to the welfare state. The authors have argued that the public health community needs to redefine the way people and communities are involved, in a way that does not erode hard-won rights.

The book presents many different ways of supporting lay people in their public health roles. Policy and practice in this field is complex and there are multiple dimensions to consider. This is rarely about neat solutions; it is more often about understanding relationships between services and communities. A number of themes have threaded throughout the book, whether critiquing policy, analysing practice or exploring contrasting perspectives on lay engagement. These themes are summarised below.

Advancing a rationale for citizen involvement in public health activity

There is a strong rationale for involving members of the public in public health programme delivery. This rationale is supported by an evidence base, underpinned by theoretical perspectives (Altpeter et al, 1998; Wallerstein, 2002; Dennis, 2003; Chiu and West, 2007), and linked to the centrality of empowerment within health promotion discourse (World Health Organization, 2009). The People in Public Health study confirmed that involving lay people in service delivery is also valued by those who have practical experience of working in this way, whether as practitioners, as lay health workers or as programme recipients.

Chapter Four set out six reasons for involving members of the public in programme delivery (see Box 12.1), based on the findings of the People in Public Health study, and also discussed some of the drawbacks identified. The justifications were further explored in the case studies of real-life projects and in Chapter Five, where lay perspectives on involvement were presented. The conclusion is that citizen involvement should be viewed as a positive strategy to add value to public health programmes and public services, as well as enhancing democracy and accountability. It is not about plugging a gap in service capacity or getting a workforce 'on the cheap' (Hongoro and McPake, 2004; Neuberger, 2008), although it is acknowledged that arguments for increasing volunteering can play into neoliberal discourses on individualism and a smaller state (see Chapter Eleven). Involving members of the public in programme delivery is about increasing reach, breaking down barriers and enhancing access to the resources that support good health. It is also about helping services tailor provision better to community needs and, ultimately, about enhancing democratic control. The bridging role of lay health workers is critical (American Association of Diabetes Educators, 2003). One of the core roles of lay health workers, whatever the setting, is to work as connectors: connecting people to services, connecting services to community intelligence, strengthening social networks and linking up to further opportunities, whether education-, health- or employment-related. It is the bridging between the professional and lay spheres that differentiates lay health worker approaches from other forms of community mobilisation, like self-help or community development.

Box 12.1: Six reasons for involving members of the public in programme delivery

1. To provide an essential bridging function, reducing barriers between services and communities, particularly where groups are at risk of social exclusion.

2. To reduce communication barriers, as lay health workers have the potential to reach some communities that professionals cannot.

3. To provide peer support to other community members to help them achieve better health.

4. To increase service capacity by having a 'community workforce' as well as a professional workforce.

5. To offer an opportunity for people to gain directly in terms of increased confidence, health literacy, self-fulfilment, social contact, skills and employability.

6. To open up a conduit so that information can be cascaded through social networks and community knowledge can be fed back up to inform strategic planning and service delivery.

Source: South et al (2010b, p 225).

Lay health workers as a strategy for tackling health inequalities

The introduction to the book set the challenge of more effective community engagement in health in the context of efforts to reduce health inequalities. Connected, resilient and, ultimately, empowered communities are a building block of health equity (The Marmot Review, 2010b). Many UK and international examples used in the book serve to demonstrate that lay health worker programmes are an effective means to reach and engage excluded or disadvantaged populations. It is important not to lose sight of the bigger question of whether the coverage and the accessibility of services are sufficient to meet health needs, as many of the international examples occur in welfare regimes that are less comprehensive than the UK welfare state. The World Health Organization (2007, p 5) states that community health worker programmes are 'neither the panacea for weak health systems nor a cheap option to provide access to health care to underserved populations'. Within the context of these broader debates about health systems, lay health workers have an important role in removing barriers for people so that they can attain the resources to which they are entitled. Involving lay people in service delivery can therefore be part of a strategic response to promote greater equity in health based on the principles of both active and social citizenship (South et al, 2011a).

This response should not be limited to making people feel more comfortable in using existing services. As Wilkinson and Pickett (2009) have eloquently argued in *The spirit level*, inequality is not just about material differences between rich and poor, it also concerns relationships, and manifests as lower levels of trust, differences in social status, low self-esteem and so on. An equitable public health system would, therefore, seek to address power imbalances and would use strategies to promote individuals' self-worth and capabilities as well as building stronger communities. Evidently, lay health workers can play an important part in this endeavour.

The impending transfer of public health to local authorities in the English public health system brings genuine opportunities to strengthen relationships with communities and to enable people to gain more control over their health and their lives (see Chapter Two). The broad remit of local authorities makes it easier to locate citizens within the socio-economic and cultural context within which they live and for public health to work with citizens to co-produce solutions that are attuned to their circumstances and aspirations. More broadly, there needs to be greater recognition of the assets within communities. In tune with a zeitgeist that is seeking alternative solutions to intractable problems, there is growing interest in asset-based approaches. In the UK, the Improvement and Development Agency publication *A glass half-full* (Foot and Hopkins, 2010) drew attention to the relevance of these approaches to public health (see Box 12.2).

Box 12.2: Asset-based approaches for public health

The UK welfare state is underpinned by a deficit model; thus, people are defined by their needs, which state services attempt to meet. While not denying that people do have needs, an asset-based approach starts from the premise that individuals and communities also have knowledge, connections, capacity and resources that can be mobilised in order to produce better health outcomes (Foot and Hopkins, 2010). Morgan and Ziglio (2007, p 18) define a 'health asset' as:

> any factor (or resource), which enhances the ability of individuals, groups, communities, populations, social systems and/or institutions to maintain and sustain health and well-being and to help to reduce health inequities. These assets can operate at the level of the individual, group, community, and/or population as protective (or promoting) factors to buffer against life's stresses.

Assets can therefore be the skills, capacity and knowledge of individuals, their interests and commitment, the social networks within communities, resources of local voluntary organisations, or the physical and economic resources within a locality (Foot and Hopkins, 2010). A range of methods can be used to harness these assets including Asset Mapping, Asset-Based Community Development (ABCD), Appreciative Inquiry and Participatory Appraisal. Asset-based approaches seek to provide an alternative perspective to deficit-based approaches that focus on population needs and problems. It is the emphasis on deficits in public health that Morgan and Ziglio (2007) argue needs rebalancing in order to address health inequalities more effectively.

While asset-based approaches are currently attracting interest in the UK, the ideas can be traced back to earlier theories. The concept of salutogenesis (Lindstrom and Erikkson, 2005), encompassing an orientation to positive health and well-being and the factors that promote resilience, underpins asset-based approaches. In the US, a strong tradition of ABCD has flourished, led by John McKnight at The Asset-Based Community Development Institute (The Asset-Based Community Development Institute, no date). ABCD offers a practical approach to community mobilisation that seeks to utilise the capabilities and capacities of individuals and voluntary associations to create community-led solutions to problems.

A 'people-centred' and 'citizen-led' approach requires widespread cultural change in the way statutory services operate (Foot and Hopkins, 2010). There is a need to question whether asset approaches can represent a shift in responsibility from the state to individuals. In the ABCD model, the balance is towards encouraging self-reliance and self-organising in communities, and moving away from what is termed welfare dependency (Kretzmann and Green, 1998; McKnight, 2009). Foot and Hopkins (2010) stress that it is about what can be done to complement, not replace, public services; nonetheless, there is a risk that in the current economic climate, community mobilisation will be used to mask deficits in statutory services. Asset-based approaches, therefore, need to work within a citizenship model that harnesses community skills, knowledge and commitment in an effective and equitable manner.

The active citizenship offer

A strong argument has been made that lay health workers are a manifestation of active citizenship. As Chapter Five shows, people come into these roles motivated primarily from a commitment to their communities and for altruistic reasons. They bring valuable skills, local knowledge and life experience. The case studies show that what happens cannot always be packaged into a neat, bounded intervention. This is about people playing a part in their communities and activities spill over from the intervention into community life. Walking for Health is a prime example of this; Chapter Six describes how the volunteer leader role helps grow the group, which becomes a mechanism to build both bridging and bonding social capital. Public services, therefore, have a role in nurturing and supporting social action, but top-heavy supervision and control could easily inhibit the very processes that are most beneficial to health. This is not about developing a semi-professional workforce, it is about respecting people's contribution and building capacity for change.

It should also be remembered that, as Chapters Two and Three discuss, active citizenship can involve action independent of professional services as well as roles within professionally determined interventions. A large proportion of people are already engaged in volunteering in the UK, many of these would not see their role as related to 'health' even if their roles (eg sports coaches or park friends) contribute to improving the environments in which people live and work. Active citizens may also challenge the status quo as part of their contribution. Social movements, like the women's health movement, are about people taking more control over their lives and their health. While the scope of the book has been limited to lay health workers, there are evident connections to citizen involvement in democratic processes, including campaigns and advocacy. Future directions include the growing link between public health and sustainable development, in which active citizens have the potential to play a major part in locally based solutions (see Box 12.3).

Box 12.3: Lay engagement for a sustainable world

Sustainable development and public health are inextricably linked, both sharing the principles of 'reducing health inequalities, promoting and protecting health, prevention of disease and prolonging life' (Wilson and Mabhala, 2009, p 74). Arguably, climate change, the result of the failure of the developed world to live sustainably, along with growing inequality are the greatest public health challenges facing society (Hunter et al, 2010) and very possibly the greatest threats facing the planet (Vidal, 2011). Tackling climate change means that people in the developed world, in particular, need to live differently. According to Schofield (no date):

> A radical restructuring of the economy around local sufficiency and security is required, where the essentials of material life, including food, housing, energy and transport are provided through local production. The short-term objective will be to minimize the throughput of energy and materials and to create a zero-carbon economy that helps stabilise climate change.

At first appearance, the argument for sustainable development may seem to have little to do with lay engagement to improve health, but if sustainable development and public health share the same principles and climate change is one of, if not the greatest threat, to public health, then common solutions should be sought. Hunter et al (2010) argue that a 'new public health movement' is needed that embraces tackling climate change and building more sustainable communities as well as addressing health inequalities. The engagement of individuals and communities is a necessary part of building such a movement and needs to be combined with action at a macro-level (driven by the grassroots) to tackle the causes of health inequalities. Action to combat climate change and build a more sustainable global world needs to be, and often is, founded not just on macro-level solutions, but on people changing the way they live and working together to become more locally sufficient.

Throughout this book, there are examples of how people are actively engaging in improving their health. There are key elements in common with the way people organise together to be more self-sufficient or to combat climate change:

- People are becoming active rather than remaining passive.
- They are finding local solutions.
- They are struggling against a system that is not used to working with empowered service users and citizens.
- They are improving their health and well-being.
- They are addressing inequalities and building a healthier, more sustainable world, from the bottom up.

> An example of where people are engaging locally to improve health and live more sustainably is in local food growing. Across the country, people are growing food in their gardens and backyards or taking on allotments and, thereby, both improving their health and well-being and reducing their carbon footprint. Where this is a group or community endeavour, it builds social capital as well as contributing to more sustainable and healthy lifestyles (see Back to Front, no date; Local Government Improvement and Development, 2009; Incredible Edible Todmorden, 2012).

Building new relationships

A theme running through the book has been the benefits of building new, more equal, relationships between services and communities. It has been argued that an instrumental approach to lay engagement, where lay health workers are used as a resource for delivery, has limited value. It fails to recognise the value of developing individuals who can broker connections and improve the bilateral flow of intelligence between communities and services. That is not to say that recruiting and training lay people to deliver standardised, professionally led interventions is in any way inappropriate. The Cardiovascular Health Awareness Program in Canada provides a powerful example of the effectiveness of integrating volunteers into a hypertension screening programme (Carter et al, 2009; Kaczorowski et al, 2011; see also Box 3.4 in Chapter Three). Even where volunteers simply 'help out', a friendly word and a cup of tea can make people comfortable enough to participate, for example, in a weight management clinic.

The aspiration to give people a greater role in public health is part of the wider challenge of developing governance systems that provide a genuine opportunity for citizen involvement in health, both at a collective and individual level. Policy development nationally and internationally is reflecting a renewed emphasis on participation, for example, within the new European health policy 'Health 2020' (World Health Organization Regional Office for Europe, 2012). The NHS Future Forum on *Patient involvement and public accountability* (NHS Future Forum, 2011b, p 4) noted that there were 'three major, inter-connecting priorities', namely:

- integrated care for patients and communities;
- embedding the voice of patients and the public in health services; and
- effective systems for accountability and governance.

In June 2012, the NHS Confederation released an important briefing titled *Community Health Champions: creating new relationships with patients and communities* (NHS Confederation and Altogether Better, 2012) (for information on community health champions, see Chapter Three). The briefing challenges NHS leaders with a series of questions:

- Are there activities you could facilitate within your local community to involve local people in co-production of their own health, care and well-being?
- Are there activities within your organisation that could be undertaken by volunteers that would enhance the quality, experience or outcomes of services, increase capacity, or reduce future demand?
- Are there local volunteer-led groups or volunteer-involving organisations that you could be working with to improve the health and well-being of the local community and engage more people in co-creating health?
- Are the voices of people from the local community, including those with health and care needs, families, carers, and volunteers being heard in the process of needs assessment? Are these voices influencing priorities for the services you commission?
- Are there services that you are responsible for commissioning in which people with health and care needs, volunteers, and members of the community play a greater part?

These questions highlight that the challenge of governance is not just about structures, it is also about relationships and recognising the contribution of lay people. The conclusion of this book is that there needs to be greater understanding of the value members of the public bring as an integral part of the public health system. Lay health worker programmes can become the basis of powerful partnerships, which have the capacity to deliver services better aligned to needs. This requires a cultural shift in the way organisations and professionals work and links to the ideas of co-production (see Box 12.4). Chapter Ten presents an example of co-production around diabetes care, with partnerships between clients, community health champions, health trainers and primary care.

Box 12.4: Co-production – creating equality between services and users

Co-production concerns the joint working between service users and professionals to produce better (health) outcomes. It is an idea whose roots can be traced back to civil rights discourse in America in the 1970s (Realpe and Wallace, 2010). More recently, co-production has been championed by organisations such as the New Economics Foundation (NEF) and National Endowment for Science, Technology and the Arts (NESTA). The facilitation of a reciprocal relationship between client and professional is the defining feature of co-production approaches (Ryan-Collins et al, 2007, p 13):

> Co-production involves sharing responsibilities and knowledge – of both service design and delivery – between professionals and users, and sometimes with the user's family and neighbours. A co-production approach recognises that everyone has assets that need to be engaged to make society work. This approach requires a relationship of reciprocity

and partnership between commissioners, providers and users that recognises each has a vital role to play in achieving the best outcomes.

Co-production approaches have been applied to the management of long-term conditions and associated with concepts such as patient-centredness, personalisation, shared decision-making and self-care (Realpe and Wallace, 2010). Its relevance to approaches described in this book lies in the recognition of the lay contribution to service delivery. Boyle et al (2006) argue that co-production extends the traditional view of volunteering because it involves redefining relationships between providers and communities and valuing greater participation in service delivery. NEF, similarly, sees it connected to a radical critique of public services based on passive consumers. It is argued that traditional models of provision fail to recognise the significance of relationships between client and professional and the social networks that support people (Ryan-Collins et al, 2007). In contrast, successful co-production projects have a number of features (Boyle et al, 2006):

- projects provide opportunities for personal growth and encourage self-organisation;
- there is investment in developing emotional intelligence for individuals and community capacity;
- peer support networks are utilised;
- boundaries between providers and recipients are blurred;
- public services adopt new roles as catalysts and facilitators; and
- a range of incentives is offered through reciprocity.

Co-production has resonance within the current policy context and there is a fit with a greater emphasis on volunteering in the context of service delivery (Boyle and Harris, 2009). Its value for public health may be in providing a model for increased citizen involvement for those using health and social care services (Boyle et al, 2010b).

A broader view of evidence

The book has highlighted the body of evidence around lay health workers and peer-based approaches. Despite the challenges of evaluating community-based interventions, especially where they involve socially excluded communities, and the need for more evidence on the impact on social networks, there is enough evidence to act. As Chapter Eleven argues, evidence is political and there needs to be greater acceptance of different types of evidence (Rada et al, 1999). There is potential for more shared learning with those with practical experience of implementing these approaches. Public health managers and practitioners cannot always prove that things work, but this does not mean that their experience is to be discounted. There is now a wealth of expertise in the UK about how to engage communities, developed through programmes like health trainers. Recently, an Active Citizens for Health network was formed to act as a think tank and as a hub for evidence and good practice.

A broader view of evidence would also incorporate lay voices. The book has attempted to redress the balance in the academic literature by directly reporting the views of lay people engaged in the case studies and other projects. More attention needs to be paid to listening to those who experience first hand the effect of health inequalities if services are to be tailored to meet needs. This requires a cultural shift away from decision-making using only evidence from well-designed experimental studies (the so-called gold standard), to acceptance of a broad range of sources of evidence, including lay perspectives.

A supportive infrastructure

If success is to be achieved in implementing and scaling up lay health worker programmes, there needs to be some acknowledgement that effective community involvement does not occur spontaneously. As the People in Public Health study showed, current systems are not really set up to involve members of the public in this way. The expert hearings held in 2008 highlighted the importance of professional support being available to facilitate individuals' participation, including inclusive recruitment strategies, training focused on personal development and ongoing support through projects (South et al, 2009). These processes are often part and parcel of how health promotion programmes work. They can be underpinned by good community development at a local level (Smithies and Webster, 1998). As discussed in Chapter Ten, professional support is not enough to grow and sustain citizen involvement; there is a need for organisational support within the public health system and a reorientation of health services (South et al, 2011c). In other words, there is a need for a supportive infrastructure that uses appropriate commissioning models, that seeks to include lay voices and increase community control, and that works for the long term, not just in short policy cycles. The type of public health system that nurtures citizen involvement in health is one that fits with the Ottawa Charter in developing personal skills, reorienting health services, creating supportive environments, strengthening community action and developing healthy public policy (World Health Organization, 1986).

The current public health system needs reform if there is to be effective action on the social determinants of health. The conclusion of this book is that individuals and communities need to be involved as part of mainstream public health action. The Marmot Review (2010a, p 152) calls for 'political, civic and managerial leadership in public services' to focus on 'creating the conditions in which people and communities take control'. As authors, we now set out a vision for a new public health system; one that incorporates the values of citizenship, reflects the learning and evidence set out in the book, and is based on the principles of health promotion.

A citizen-centred public health system

- Citizens need to be the centre of the public health system. A culture change is required to shift from a deficit- to an asset-based approach that recognises the contribution that can be made by people in the places where they live and work.
- Public health action should shift from an outdated biomedical model still focused on health behaviours and targets, to addressing the social determinants that impact on people's lives in line with the Rio Declaration (World Health Organization, 2011) and the recommendations of The Marmot Review (2010a).
- Professionals and policymakers cannot sort this out on their own, involving communities only as an afterthought as part of targeted interventions. The public health system should create the space for a bottom-up social movement on health. A healthy society is one with strong, connected communities who are able to participate in decisions about their health.
- The public health system needs to be more joined up so that citizen involvement can make a difference across different aspects of social life. Commissioning in silos is not going to provide the investment in community capacity-building that is needed. Commissioning models need to take account of the wider health and social benefits that can result from citizen involvement.
- Public health capacity can be increased by enabling and supporting the public to become more involved. Lay heath workers and volunteers can add value to mainstream service provision. The focus should be on enhancing people's confidence and capacity to take on a public health role, not on producing a new layer of semi-professionalised workers.
- A supportive infrastructure needs to be in place to nurture citizen involvement. Involvement should be well resourced and supported so lay capacity adds value, people's experiences are positive and turnover is reduced.
- Leadership is needed to advocate for a citizen-centred public health system. This needs to happen in national policymaking, but also in local health systems.
- Citizenship is about democracy and it is about rights. Involving members of the public in public health should not be about reducing public services. It is a way of reducing barriers to the resources that support good health and should be framed as a strategy to increase equity in health.

In conclusion, the book has set out to challenge traditional ideas on lay engagement and present fresh perspectives on why and how public health can successfully harness people power. The arguments for increasing volunteering and building lay health worker programmes are set against a backdrop of the economic, social and political challenges faced by society. This is a time when the old certainties are being challenged, including in public health. The book ends with a radical vision of how public health might be done differently. This would involve creating a new professional culture, strong partnerships with communities, a robust and supportive infrastructure, and a broad evidence base. This is a citizenship model where rights and responsibilities around health are in balance.

References

Abbatt, F. (2005) *Scaling up health and education workers: community health workers*, London: DFID Health Systems Resource Centre.

Acheson, D. (1998) *Independent inquiry into inequalities in health*, London: The Stationery Office.

Altogether Better (no date) 'Homepage'. Available at: http://www.altogetherbetter.org.uk/

Altogether Better (2010) *Altogether Better Programme: phase 1 development*, Leeds: Altogether Better, Big Lottery Fund.

Altogether Better Regional Programme Team (2009) *Altogether Better Programme executive summary, 2008/9*, Leeds: Altogether Better.

Altpeter, M., Earp, J.L. and Schopler, J.H. (1998) 'Promoting breast cancer screening in rural African American communities: the "science and art" of community health promotion', *Health & Social Work*, vol 23, no 2, pp 104–15.

American Association of Diabetes Educators (2003) 'Diabetes community health workers', *The Diabetes Educator*, vol 29, no 5, pp 818–24.

Amos, M. (2002) 'Community development', in Adams, L., Amos, M. and Munro, J. (eds) *Promoting health: politics and practice*, London: Sage, pp 63–71.

Andrews, J.O., Felton, G., Wewers, M.E. and Heath, J. (2004) 'Use of community health workers in research with ethnic minority women', *Journal of Nursing Scholarship*, vol 36, no 4, pp 358–65.

Attree, P. (2004) '"It was like my little acorn, and it's going to grow into a big tree": a qualitative study of a community support project', *Health and Social Care in the Community*, vol 12, no 2, pp 155–161.

Back To Front (no date) 'Homepage'. Available at: http://www.backtofront.org.uk/

Bagnall, A.-M. (2009) 'The people in public health database', Leeds Metropolitan University. Available at: https://piph.leedsmet.ac.uk/main/litreview.htm

Bailey, T.M., Delva, J., Gretebeck, K., Siefert, K. and Ismail, A. (2005) 'A systematic review of mammography educational interventions for low-income women', *American Journal of Health Promotion*, vol 20, no 2, pp 96–107.

Baines, S. and Hardill, I. (2008) '"At least I can do something": the work of volunteering in a community beset by worklessness', *Social Policy and Society*, vol 7, no 3, pp 307–17.

Ball, S.J. (2007) 'Big policies/small world: an introduction to international perspectives in education policy', in Lingard, B. and Ozga, J. (eds) *The RoutledgeFalmer reader in education policy and politics*, Oxon: Routledge, pp 36–47.

Bambra, C., Fox, D. and Scott-Samuel, A. (2005) 'Towards a politics of health', *Health Promotion International*, vol 20, no 2, pp 187–93.

Banks, S. (2003) 'The concept of "community practice"', in Banks, S., Butcher, H., Henderson, P. and Robertson, J. (eds) *Managing community practice. Principles, policies, and programmes*, Bristol: The Policy Press, pp 7–22.

Barnes, C. and Mercer, G. (eds) (2006) *Independent futures: creating user-led disability services in a disabling society*, Bristol: The Policy Press.

Barr, A. (2003) 'Participative planning and evaluation skills', in Banks, S., Butcher, H., Henderson, P. and Robertson, J. (eds) *Managing community practice. Principles, policies, and programmes*, Bristol: The Policy Press, pp 137–53.

Barr, A. and Hashagen, S. (2000) *ABCD handbook. A framework for evaluating community development*, London: Community Development Foundation.

Bauld, L. and Judge, K. (eds) (2002) *Learning from Health Action Zones*, Chichester: Aeneas Press.

Beresford, P. (2001) 'Service users, social policy and the future of welfare', *Critical Social Policy*, vol 21, no 4, pp 494–512.

Berrios, C. (2002) 'A look at certifcation for promotores(as)', *Migrant Health Newsline*, vol 19, no 4, pp 1–2.

Bhutta, Z.A., Lassi, Z.A., Pariyo, G. and Huicho, L. (2010) *Global experience of community health workers for delivery of health related Millenium Development Goals: a systematic review, country case studies, and recommendations for integration into national health systems*, Geneva: World Health Organization, Global Health Workforce Alliance.

Billis, D. and Glennerster, H. (1998) 'Human services and the voluntary sector: towards a theory of comparative advantage', *Journal of Social Policy*, vol 27, no 1, pp 70–98.

Blond, P. (ed) (2010) *Red Tory: how Left and Right have broken Britain and how we can fix it*, London: Faber and Faber.

Blunkett, D. (2003) *Active citizens, strong communities. Progressing civic renewal*, London: Home Office.

Bolton, M. (no date) *Voluntary sector added value: A discussion paper*, London: National Council for Voluntary Organisations (NCVO).

Borgonovi, F. (2008) 'Doing well by doing good. The relationship between formal volunteering and self-reported health and happiness', *Social Science and Medicine*, vol 66, no 11, pp 2321–34.

Bosley, S. and Dale, J. (2008) 'Healthcare assistants in general practice: practical and conceptual issues of skill-mix change', *British Journal of General Practice*, vol 58, no 547, pp 118–24.

Boyle, D. and Harris, M. (2009) *The challenge of co-production: how equal partnerships between professionals and the public are crucial to improving public services*, London: National Endowment for Science, Technology and the Arts, New Economics Foundation.

Boyle, D., Clark, S. and Burns, S. (2006) *Hidden work. Co-production by people outside paid employment*, York: Joseph Rowntree Foundation.

Boyle, D., Coote, A., Sherwood, C. and Slay, J. (2010a) *Right here, right now: taking co-production into the mainstream*, London: National Endowment for Science, Technology and the Arts.

Boyle, D., Slay, J. and Stephens, L. (2010b) *Public services inside out: putting co-production into practice*, London: National Endowment for Science, Technology and the Arts, New Economics Foundation.

Bracht, N. and Tsouros, A. (1990) 'Principles and strategies of effective participation', *Health Promotion International*, vol 5, no 3, pp 199–208.

Bradley, P. (2007) *Antisocial Britain and the challenge of citizenship*, London: Social Market Foundation.

Bridgen, P. (2004) 'Evaluating the empowering potential of community-based health schemes: the case of community health policies in the UK since 1997', *Community Development Journal*, vol 39, no 3, pp 289–302.

Britten, J., Hoddinott, P. and Mcinnes, R. (2006) 'Breastfeeding peer support: health service programmes in Scotland', *British Journal of Midwifery*, vol 14, no 1, pp 12–19. (Corrected: published erratum appears in [2006] *British Journal of Midwifery*, vol 14, no 4, p 232.)

Brooks, K. (2002) 'Talking about volunteering: a discourse analysis approach to volunteer motivations', *Voluntary Action. The Journal for the Institute of Volunteering Research*, vol 4, no 3, pp 13–29.

Brown, P. and Zavestoski, S. (eds) (2005) *Social movements in health*, Oxford: Blackwell.

Brownstein, J.N., Chowdhury, F.M., Norris, S.L., Horsley, T., Jack, L., Zhang, X. and Satterfield, D. (2007) 'Effectiveness of community health workers in the care of people with hypertension', *American Journal of Preventive Medicine*, vol 32, no 5, pp 435–47.

Burton, P. (2009) 'Conceptual, theoretical and practical issues in measuring the benefits of public participation', *Evaluation*, vol 15, no 3, pp 263–84.

Butcher, H. (1993) 'Introduction: some examples and definitions', in Butcher, H., Glen, A., Henderson, P. and Smith, J. (eds) *Community and public policy*, London: Pluto Press, pp 3–21.

Cabinet Office (2010) 'Building the Big Society'. Available at: http://www.cabinetoffice.gov.uk/sites/default/files/resources/building-big-society_0.pdf

Cabinet Office (2011) 'Big Society – overview'. Available at: http://www.cabinetoffice.gov.uk/content/big-society-overview

Cameron, D. (2011) 'PM's speech on Big Society', British Prime Minister's Office. Available at: http://www.number10.gov.uk/news/pms-speech-on-big-society/

Campbell, F., Hughes, L. and Gilling, T. (2008) *Reaching out: community engagement and health*, London: Improvement and Development Agency (IDeA).

Carlisle, S. (2000) 'Health promotion, advocacy and health inequalities: a conceptual framework', *Health Promotion International*, vol 15, no 4, pp 369–76.

Carr, S.M., Clarke, C.L., Molyneaux, J. and Jones, D. (2006) 'Facilitating participation: a Health Action Zone experience', *Primary Health Care Research and Development*, vol 7, no 2, pp 147–56.

Carter, M., Karwalajtys, T., Chambers, L., Kaczorowski, J., Dolovich, L., Gierman, T., Cross, D. and Laryea, S. (2009) 'Implementing a standardized community-based cardiovascular risk assessment program in 20 Ontario communities', *Health Promotion International*, vol 24, no 4, pp 325–33.

Casiday, R., Kinsman, E., Fisher, C. and Bambra, C. (2008) *Volunteering and health; what impact does it really have?*, London: Volunteering England.

Centers for Disease Control and Prevention (2003) *Community health workers/ Promotores de salud: critical connections in communities*, Atlanta, GA: Centers for Disease Control and Prevention Division of Diabetes Translation.

CHAP (Cardiovascular Health Awareness Program) (2009) 'Current CHAP results', *Connections*, Autumn. Available at: http://www.chapprogram.ca/publications_newsletters/newsletters/autumn2009main/document_view

Chiu, L.F. (2003) *Application and management of the Community Health Educator model. A handbook for practitioners*, Leeds: Nuffield Institute for Health.

Chiu, L.F. and West, R. (2007) 'Health intervention in social context: understanding social networks and neighbourhood', *Social Science and Medicine*, vol 65, pp 1915–27.

Citizen Foundation (2012) 'What is citizenship?'. Available at: http://www.citizenshipfoundation.org.uk/main/page.php?427

Collica, K. (2002) 'Levels of knowledge and risk perceptions about HIV/AIDS among female inmates in New York State: can prison-based HIV programs set the stage for behavior change?', *The Prison Journal*, vol 82, pp 101–24.

Commissioning Support Programme and Kindle (2010) *Commissioning and the Big Society: the role of the community sector*, UK: Commissioning Support Programme, Kindle.

Communities and Local Government (2007) *An action plan for community empowerment: building on success*, London: Communities and Local Government.

Community Health Exchange (no date) 'What we do'. Available at: http://www.chex.org.uk/what-we-do/

Community Sector Coalition (2010) *Unseen, unequal, untapped, unleashed: the potential for community action at the grassroots*, London: Community Sector Coalition.

Conrad, P. (1992) 'Medicalization and social control', *Annual Review of Sociology*, vol 18, pp 209–32.

Cooksey, D. (2006) *A review of UK health research funding*, London: HM Treasury.

Cooper, C., Arber, F.L. and Ginn, J. (1999) *The Influence of social support and social capital on health*, London: Health Education Authority.

Coote, A. (2010) *Cutting it. The 'Big Society' and the new austerity*, London: New Economics Foundation.

Corluka, A., Walker, D.G., Lewin, S.A., Glenton, C. and Scheel, I.B. (2009) 'Are vaccination programmes delivered by lay health workers cost-effective? A systematic review', *Human Resources for Health*, vol 7, no 81, doi:10.1186/1478-4491-7-81.

Cornwall, A. (2008) 'Unpacking "participation": models, meanings and practices', *Community Development Journal*, vol 43, no 3, pp 269–83.

Coufopoulos, A., Coffey, M. and Dugdill, L. (2010) 'Working as a community food worker: voices from the inside', *Perspectives in Public Health*, vol 130, no 4, pp 180–5.

Cowden, S. and Singh, G. (2007) 'The "user": friend, foe or fetish? A critical exploration of user involvement in health and social care', *Critical Social Policy*, vol 27, pp 15–23.

Crisp, N. (2010) *Turning the world upside down – the search for global health in the 21st century*, London: Hodder Education.

Curtis, P., Woodhill, R. and Stapleton, H. (2007) 'The peer–professional interface in a community-based, breast feeding peer-support project', *Midwifery*, vol 23, no 2, pp 146–56.

CutsWatch (2012) 'Homepage'. Available at: http://www.cutswatch.org.uk/main/

Daley, A. (2006) 'Lesbian and gay health issues: OUTside of Canada's health policy', *Critical Social Policy*, vol 26, no 4, pp 794–816.

Davies, B. (2003) 'Death to critique and dissent? The policies and practices of new managerialism and of "evidence-based practice"', *Gender and Education*, vol 15, pp 91–103.

Davies, J. (2009) 'Zapatista healthcare advances'. Available at: http://narcosphere.narconews.com/notebook/jessica-davies/2009/03/zapatista-healthcare-advances

Davies, R. and Mitchell, L. (2008) *Building bridges: philanthropy strengthening communities*, London: Policy Exchange.

Dennis, C. (2002) 'Breastfeeding peer support: maternal and volunteer perceptions from a randomized controlled trial', *Birth: Issues in Perinatal Care*, vol 29, no 3, pp 169–76.

Dennis, C.-L. (2003) 'Peer support within a healthcare context: a concept analysis', *International Journal of Nursing Studies*, vol 40, no 3, pp 321–32.

Department for Communities and Local Government (2011) *Community action in England: a report on the 2009–10 citizenship survey*, London: Department for Communities and Local Government.

Department for Education and Skills (2002) *Sure Start. Making a difference for children and families*, London: DfES.

Department of Health (no date) 'Introduction to the skills escalator'. Available at: http://webarchive.nationalarchives.gov.uk/+/www.dh.gov.uk/en/Managingyourorganisation/Humanresourcesandtraining/Modelcareer/DH_405552

Department of Health (1999) 'Health Action Zones in £78 million trailblazing of money for modernisation', press release 1999/0034, London: Department of Health.

Department of Health (2001a) *The expert patient: a new approach to chronic disease management for the 21st century*, London: Department of Health.

Department of Health (2001b) *Involving patients and the public in healthcare. A discussion document*, London: Department of Health.

Department of Health (2001c) *The report of the Chief Medical Officer's project to strengthen the public health function*, London: Department of Health.

Department of Health (2001d) *Shifting the balance of power. Securing delivery*, London: Department of Health.

Department of Health (2002) *Shifting the balance of power: the next steps*, London: Department of Health.

Department of Health (2003) *Tackling health inequalities: a programme for action*, London: Department of Health.

Department of Health (2004) *Choosing health. Making healthier choices easier*, London: The Stationery Office.

Department of Health (2005a) *Delivering 'Choosing health': making healthier choices easier*, London: Department of Health.

Department of Health (2005b) *'Now I feel tall'. What a patient-led NHS feels like*, London: COI.

Department of Health (2006) *Best research for best health: a new national health research strategy*, London: Department of Health.

Department of Health (2007) *World Class Commissioning: competencies*, London: Department of Health.

Department of Health (2008a) *Health inequalities: progress and next steps*, London: Department of Health.

Department of Health (2008b) *Towards a strategy to support volunteering in health and social care: consultation*, London: Department of Health.

Department of Health (2009) *Be active, be healthy: a plan for getting the nation active*, London: Department of Health.

Department of Health (2010a) *The framework for NHS involvement in international development*, London: Department of Health.

Department of Health (2010b) 'Health trainers – review to date – February 2010'. Available at: http://www.healthtrainersengland.com/about-health-trainers

Department of Health (2010c) *A vision for adult social care: capable communities and active citizens*, London: Department of Health.

Department of Health (2011a) *Healthy lives, healthy people. Summary of responses to the consultations on our strategy for public health in England*, London: Department of Health.

Department of Health (2011b) *Social action for health and well-being: building co-operative communities, Department of Health strategic vision for volunteering*, London: Department of Health.

Devilly, G.J., Sorbello, L., Eccleston, L. and Ward, T. (2005) 'Prison-based peer-education schemes', *Aggression and Violent Behaviour*, vol 10, no 2, pp 219–40.

Dickson-Gómez, J., Knowlton, A. and Latkin, C. (2003) 'Hoppers and oldheads: qualitative evaluation of a volunteer AIDS outreach intervention', *AIDS & Behavior*, vol 7, no 3, pp 303–15.

Dingle, A. and Heath, J. (2001) 'Volunteering matters – or does it? A UK parliamentary study of the role of voluntary action in the twenty-first century', *Voluntary Action*, vol 3, pp 11–25.

Dolan, P., Hallsworth, M., Halpern, D., King, D. and Vlaev, I. (2010) *MINDSPACE: influencing behaviour through public policy*, London: Institute for Government and Cabinet Office.

Dykes, F. (2005) 'Government funded breastfeeding peer support projects: implications for practice', *Maternal & Child Nutrition*, vol 1, no 1, pp 21–31.

Edinburgh Chiapas Solidarity Group (2011) 'Autonomous health promotion in the Zapatista communities'. Available at: http://www.edinchiapas.org.uk/node/353

El Ansari, W., Phillips, C.J. and Zwi, A.B. (2002) 'Narrowing the gap between academic professional wisdom and community lay knowledge: perceptions from partnerships', *Public Health*, vol 116, no 3, pp 151–9.

Elford, J., Sherr, L., Bolding, G., Serle, F. and Maguire, M. (2002) 'Peer-led HIV prevention among gay men in London: process evaluation', *AIDS Care*, vol 14, no 3, pp 351–60.

Eng, E. and Smith, J. (1995) 'Natural helping functions of Lay Health Advisers in breast-cancer education', *Breast Cancer Research and Treatment*, vol 35, no 1, pp 23–9.

Eng, E., Parker, E. and Harlan, C. (1997) 'Lay health advisor intervention strategies: a continuum from natural helping to paraprofessional helping', *Health Education & Behavior*, vol 24, no 4, pp 413–17.

Expert Patients Programme (2011) 'Homepage'. Available at: http://www. expertpatients.co.uk/

Faculty of Public Health (2012) 'What is public health'. Available at: http://www. fph.org.uk/what_is_public_health

Farquhar, S.A., Wiggins, N., Michael, Y.L., Luhr, G., Jordan, J. and Lopez, A. (2008) '"Sitting in different chairs": roles of the community health workers in the Poder es Salud/Power for Health Project', *Education for Health*, vol 21, no 2, p 39.

Farrant, F. and Levenson, J. (2002) *Barred citizens: volunteering and active citizenship by prisoners*, London: Prison Reform Trust.

Faulkner, M. (2005) 'Social support in the healthcare setting: the role of volunteers', *Health and Social Care in the Community*, vol 13, no 1, pp 38–45.

Fernandez, M.I., Bowen, G.S., Gay, C.L., Mattson, T.R., Bital, E. and Kelly, J.A. (2003) 'HIV, sex, and social change: applying ESID principles to HIV prevention research', *American Journal of Community Psychology*, vol 32, nos 3/4, pp 333–44.

Feuerstein, M.T. (1986) *Partners in evaluation. Evaluating development and community programmes with participants*, London: TALC, Macmillan.

Finn, D. and Simmonds, D. (2003) *Intermediate labour markets in Britain and an international review of transitional employment programmes*, London: Department for Work and Pensions.

Flax, V.L. and Earp, J.L. (1999) 'Counseled women's perspectives on their interactions with lay health advisors: a feasibility study', *Health Education Research*, vol 14, no 1, pp 15–24.

Fleury, J., Keller, C., Perez, A. and Lee, S.M. (2009) 'The role of lay health advisors in cardiovascular risk reduction: a review', *American Journal of Community Psychology*, vol 44, nos 1/2, pp 28–42.

Foot, J. and Hopkins, T. (2010) *A glass half-full: how an asset approach can improve community health and well-being*, London: Improvement and Development Agency Healthy Communities Team.

Foster, G., Taylor, S.J. C., Eldridge, S.E., Ramsay, J. and Griffiths, C.J. (2007) 'Self-management education programmes by lay leaders for people with chronic conditions', *Cochrane Database of Systematic Reviews*, vol 4, no CD005108.

Foster-Fishman, P.G., Pierce, S.J. and Van Egeren, L.A. (2009) 'Who participates and why: building a process model of citizen participation', *Health Education & Behavior*, vol 36, no 3, pp 550–69.

Foucault, M. (ed) (1977) *Discipline and punish: the birth of the prison*, New York, NY: Vintage Books.

Frankel, S. and Doggett, M. (eds) (1992) *The community health worker: effective programmes for developing countries*, Oxford: Oxford University Press.

Frankham, J. (1998) 'Peer education: the unauthorised version', *British Educational Research Journal*, vol 24, no 2, pp 179–93.

Freire, P. (ed) (1970) *Pedagogy of the oppressed*, London: Penguin.

French, R., Power, R. and Mitchell, S. (2000) 'An evaluation of peer-led STD/HIV prevention work in a public sex environment', *AIDS Care*, vol 12, no 2, pp 225–34.

Friedli, L. (2009) *Mental health, resilience and inequalities*, Denmark: World Health Organization Europe.

Gamsu, M. (2011) *Tell us what the problem is and we'll try to help – Towards more effective commissioning of local voluntary sector organisations*, Manchester: Voluntary Sector North West Regional Voices.

Gaskin, K. (2003) *A choice blend: what volunteers want from organisation and management*, London: Institute for Volunteering Research.

Gaskin, K. (2006a) *On the safe side. Risk, risk management and volunteering*, London: Volunteering England, Institute of Volunteering Research.

Gaskin, K. (2006b) *Risk toolkit. How to take care of risk in volunteering. A guide for organisations*, London: Insitute for Volunteering Research, Volunteering England.

Godlee, F. (2010) 'Are we at risk of being at risk?', *British Medical Journal*, vol 341, no c4766.

Green, J. and Tones, K. (1999) 'Towards a secure evidence base for health promotion', *Journal of Public Health Medicine*, vol 21, no 2, pp 133–9.

Griffiths, C.J., Foster, G., Ramsay, J., Eldridge, S.E. and Taylor, D. (2007) 'How effective are expert patient (lay led) education programmes for chronic disease?', *British Medical Journal*, vol 334, pp 1254–6.

Grinstead, O.A., Zack, B., Faigeles, B., Grossman, N. and Blea, L. (1999) 'Reducing postrelease HIV risk among male prison inmates: a peer led intervention', *Criminal Justice and Behavior*, vol 26, no 4, pp 453–65.

Hainsworth, J. and Barlow, J. (2003) 'The training experiences of older, volunteer lay leaders on an arthritis self-management course', *Health Education Journal*, vol 62, no 3, pp 266–77.

Hardill, I., Baines, S. and Perri, 6 (2007) 'Volunteering for all? Explaining patterns of volunteering and identifying strategies to promote it', *Policy and Politics*, vol 35, no 3, pp 395–412.

Hart, G.J. (1998) 'Peer education and community based HIV prevention for homosexual men: peer led, evidence based, or fashion driven?', *Sexually Transmitted Infections*, vol 74, no 2, pp 87–9.

Hart, J.T. (1971) 'The Inverse Care Law', *The Lancet*, i, pp 405–12.

Hawe, P. (1994) 'Capturing the meaning of "community" in community intervention evaluation: some contributions from community psychology', *Health Promotion International*, vol 9, no 3, pp 199–210.

Hawkins, S. and Restall, M. (2006) *Volunteers across the NHS: improving the patient experience and creating a patient-led service*, London: Volunteering England.

Health Trainers England (no date) 'Offender settings'. Available at: http://www.healthtrainersengland.com/prisons

Healthy Living Network Leeds (2010) 'Community Health Educators; free training', flier, Leeds: NHS Leeds.

Heggenhougen, K., Vaughan, P., Muhondwa, E. and Rutabunzibwa-Ngaiza, J. (1987) *Community health workers: the Tanzanian experience*, Oxford: Oxford University Press.

Heller, R.F., Heller, T.D. and Pattison, S. (2003) 'Putting the public back into public health. Part 1. A redefinition of public health', *Public Health*, vol 117, no 1, pp 62–5.

Helm, T. and Asthana, A. (2010) 'Unemployed told: do four weeks of unpaid work or lose your benefits', *The Observer*, 7 November.

Heron, C. and Bradshaw, G. (2010) *Walk this way: recognising value in active health prevention*, London: Local Government Information Unit and Natural England.

Hills, D., Elliott, E., Kowarzik, U., Sullivan, F., Stern, E., Platt, S., Boydell, L., Popay, J., Williams, G., Petticrew, M., Mcgregor, M., Russell, S., Wilkinson, E., Rugkasa, J., Gibson, M. and Mcdaid, D. (2007) *The evaluation of the Big Lottery Fund Healthy Living Centres Programme. Final report*, London: Bridge consortium, Big Lottery Fund.

HM Treasury (2002) *The role of the voluntary and community sector in service delivery*, London: The Stationery Office.

HM Treasury and Cabinet Office (2007) *The future role of the third sector in social and economic regeneration: final report*, London: The Stationery Office.

Hobsbawm, E.J. (ed) (1984) *Worlds of Labour: Further Studies in the History of Labour*, London: Weidenfeld and Nicolson.

Hogg, C. (ed) (1999) *Patients, power and politics. From patients to citizens*, London: Sage.

Home-Start (no date) 'Homepage'. Available at: http://www.home-start.org.uk/homepage

Hongoro, C. and Mcpake, B. (2004) 'How to bridge the gap in human resources for health', *Lancet*, vol 364, pp 1451–6.

House of Commons Health Committee (2009) *Health inequalities. Third report of session 2008–09*, HC 286–I, London: The Stationery Office.

Hudson, J. and Lowe, S. (eds) (2009) *Understanding the policy process. 2nd edition*, Bristol: The Policy Press.

Hunter, D.J. (2011) 'Is the Big Society a big con?', *Journal of Public Health*, vol 33, no 1, pp 13–14.

Hunter, D.J., Marks, L. and Smith, K.E. (2010) *The public health system in England*, Bristol: The Policy Press.

Hunter, G. and Power, R. (2002) 'Involving *Big Issue* vendors in a peer education initiative to reduce drug-related harm: a feasibility study', *Drugs: Education, Prevention & Policy*, vol 9, no 1, pp 57–69.

Illich, I. (ed) (1975) *Medical nemesis*, London: Calder & Boyars.

Imison, C., Naylor, C., Goodwin, N., Buck, D., Curry, N., Addicott, R. and Zollinger-Read, P. (2011) *Transforming our health care system: ten priorities for commissioners*, London: The King's Fund.

Incredible Edible Todmorden (2012) 'Homepage'. Available at: http://www.incredible-edible-todmorden.co.uk/

Institute for Volunteering Research and Volunteering England (2007) *Volunteering works: volunteering and social policy*, London: Institute For Volunteering Research, Volunteering England.

Institute of Economic Affairs (2010) 'About us'. Available at: http://www.iea.org.uk/about

IPSOS Mori (2011) *Natural England Walking for Health evaluation*, London: Natural England.

Irish Mexico Group (2001) 'Why are the Zapatistas different?', *Chiapas Revealed*. Available at: http://struggle.ws/pdfs/revealed.pdf

Jackson, E.J. and Parks, C.P. (1997) 'Recruitment and training issues from selected lay health advisor programs among African Americans: a 20-year perspective', *Health Education & Behavior*, vol 24, no 4, pp 418–31.

Janz, N.K., Zimmerman, M.A., Wren, P.A., Israel, B.A., Freudenberg, N. and Carter, R.J. (1996) 'Evaluation of 37 AIDS prevention projects: successful approaches and barriers to program effectiveness', *Health Education Quarterly*, vol 23, no 1, pp 80–97.

Jauffret-Roustide, M. (2009) 'Self-support for drug users in the context of harm reduction policy: a lay expertise defined by drug users' life skills and citizenship', *Health Sociology Review*, vol 18, no 2, pp 159–72.

Jones, J.A. and Owen, N. (1998) 'Neighbourhood walk: a local community-based program to promote physical activity among older adults', *Health Promotion Journal of Australia*, vol 8, no 2, pp 145–7.

Kaczorowski, J., Chambers, L.W., Dolovich, L., Paterson, J.M., Karwalajtys, T., Gierman, T., Farrell, B., Mcdonough, B., Thabane, L., Tu, K., Zagorski, B., Goeree, R., Levitt, C.A., Hogg, W., Laryea, S., Carter, M.A., Cross, D. and Sabaldt, R.J. (2011) 'Improving cardiovascular health at population level: 39 community cluster randomised trial of Cardiovascular Health Awareness Program (CHAP)', *British Medical Journal*, vol 342, no d442.

Kelly, J.A. (2004) 'Popular opinion leaders and HIV prevention peer education: resolving discrepant findings, and implications for the development of effective community programmes', *AIDS Care*, vol 16, no 2, pp 139–50.

Kelly, J.A., St. Lawrence, J.S., Stevenson, L.Y., Hauth, A.C., Kalichman, S.C., Diaz, Y.E., Brasfield, T.L., Koob, J.J. and Morgan, M.G. (1992) 'Community AIDS/HIV risk reduction: the effects of endorsements by popular people in three cities', *American Journal of Public Health*, vol 82, no 11, pp 1483–9.

Kelly, M., Swann, C., Killoran, A., Naidoo, B., Barnett-Paige, E. and Morgan, A. (2002) 'Methodological problems in constructing the evidence base in public health', Methodology Reference Group, Public Health Evidence Steering Group, Health Development Agency. Available at: http://www.nice.org.uk/aboutnice/whoweare/aboutthehda/evidencebase/keypapers/methodologiesandcriteria/starter_paper_methodological_problems_in_constructing_the_evidence_base_in_public_health.jsp

Kennedy, A., Rogers, A. and Gately, C. (2005a) 'Assessing the introduction of the expert patients programme into the NHS: a realistic evaluation of recruitment to a national lay-led self-care scheme', *Primary Health Care Research and Development*, vol 6, pp 137–48.

Kennedy, A., Rogers, A. and Gately, C. (2005b) 'From patients to providers: prospects for self-care skills trainers in the National Health Service', *Health and Social Care in the Community*, vol 13, no 5, pp 431–40.

Kennedy, L., Milton, B. and Bundred, P. (2008a) 'Lay food and health worker involvement in community nutrition and dietetics in England: roles, responsibilities and relationships with professionals', *Journal of Human Nutrition and Dietetics*, vol 21, no 3, pp 210–24.

Kennedy, L., Milton, B. and Bundred, P. (2008b) 'Lay food and health worker involvement in community nutrition and dietetics in England: definitions from the field', *Journal of Human Nutrition and Dietetics*, vol 21, pp 196–209.

Kime, N., South, J. and Lowcock, D. (2008) *An evaluation of the Bradford District Health Trainers Programme – Phase 2*, Leeds: Centre for Health Promotion Research, Leeds Metropolitan University.

Kinsella, K., South, J. and Khan, S. (2009) *HAAMLA support and information for black and minority ethnic women in Leeds. Summary report*, Leeds: Centre for Health promotion Research, Leeds Metropolitan Promotion Research, The Haamla Service, Hamara, The Leeds Teaching Hospital Trust.

Kozart, M. (2007) 'Direct democracy and health care in Zapatista land: a doctor's experience on the day of political transition'. Available at: http://www.chiapas-support.org/health.htm

Kretzmann, J.P. and Green, M.B. (1998) *Building the bridge from client to citizen: a community toolbox for welfare reform*, Evanston, IL: The Asset-Based Community Development Institute.

Kuznetsova, D. (2012) *Healthy places. Councils leading on public health*, London: New Local Government Network.

Lam, T.K., Mcphee, S.J., Mock, J., Wong, C., Doan, H.T., Nguyen, T., Lai, K.Q., Ha-Iaconis, T. and Luong, T.-N. (2003) 'Encouraging Vietnamese-American women to obtain Pap tests through lay health worker outreach and media education', *Journal of General Internal Medicine*, vol 18, no 7, pp 516–24.

Lamb, S.E., Bartlett, H.P., Ashley, A. and Bird, W. (2002) 'Can lay-led walking programmes increase physical activity in middle aged adults? A randomised controlled trial', *Journal of Epidemiology and Community Health*, vol 56, no 4, pp 246–52.

Laverack, G. (ed) (2004) *Health promotion practice: power and empowerment*, London: Sage.

Leaman, M., Lechner, C. and Sheeshka, J. (1997) 'Perspectives in practice. The Community Nutrition Worker Project: a retrospective survey of peer educators', *Journal of the Canadian Dietetic Association*, vol 58, no 1, pp 34–8.

Ledwith, M. (ed) (2005) *Community development: a critical approach*, Bristol: The Policy Press.

Lehmann, U. and Sanders, D. (2007) *Community health workers: what do we know about them? The state of the evidence on programmes, activities, costs and impact on health outcomes of using community health workers*, Geneva: World Health Organization.

Levenson, R. and Gillam, S. (1998) *Linkworkers in primary care*, London: King's Fund.

Lewin, S.A., Dick, J., Pond, P., Zwarenstein, M., Aja, G., Van Wyk, B., Bosch-Capblanch, X. and Patrick, M. (2005) 'Lay health workers in primary and community health care', *Cochrane Database of Systematic Reviews*, issue 1, CD004015.

Lewin, S.A., Lewin, S.A., Babigumira, S.M., Bosch-Capblanch, X., Aja, G., Van Wyk, B., Glenton, C., Scheel, I., Zwarenstein, M. and Daniels, K. (2006) *Lay health workers in primary and community care: a systematic review of trials*, London: London School of Hygiene and Tropical Medicine.

Lewin, S.A., Munabi-Babigumira, S., Glenton, C., Daniels, K., Bosch-Capblanch, X. and Van Wyk, B. (2010) 'Lay health workers in primary and community health care for maternal and child health and management of infectious diseases', *Cochrane Database of Systematic Reviews*, issue 3, CD004015.

Lindström, B. and Eriksson, M. (2005) 'Salutogenesis', *Journal of Epidemiology and Community Health*, vol 59, pp 440–2.

Local Government Improvement and Development (2009) 'Middlesbrough – Berwick Hills allotments'. Available at: http://www.idea.gov.uk/idk/core/page.do?pageId=14103157

Love, M.B., Legion, V., Shim, J.K., Tsai, C., Quijano, V. and Davis, C. (2004) 'CHWs get credit: a 10-year history of the first college-credit certificate for community health workers in the United States', *Health Promotion Practice*, vol 5, no 4, pp 418–28.

Low, N., Butt, S., Ellis Paine, A. and Davis Smith, J. (2008) *Helping out. A national survey of volunteering and charitable giving*, London: Cabinet Office, Office of the Third Sector.

Maginn, B. (ed) (2010) *Total neighbourhood. Placing power back into the community*, London: Localis.

Mason, A.R., Carr Hill, R., Myers, L.A. and Street, A.D. (2008) 'Establishing the economics of engaging communities in health promotion: what is desirable, what is feasible?', *Critical Public Health*, vol 18, no 3, pp 285–97.

McKee, M. and Raine, R. (2005) 'Chosing health? First choose your philosophy', *The Lancet*, vol 365, pp 369–71.

McKee, M., Hurst, L., Aldridge, R.W., Raine, R., Mindell, J.S., Wolfe, I. and Holland, W.W. (2011) 'Public health in England: an option for the way forward?', *The Lancet*, vol 378, pp 536–9.

McKnight, J. (2009) 'Community capacities and community necessities', Clients to Citizens Forum, Coady International Institute, St. Francis Xavier University, Antigonish, Nova Scotia.

McQueen, D. (2001) 'Strengthening the evidence base for health promotion', *Health Promotion International*, vol 16, no 3, pp 261–8.

McQuiston, C. and Uribe, L. (2001) 'Latino recruitment and retention strategies: community-based HIV prevention', *Journal of Immigrant Health*, vol 3, no 2, pp 97–105.

Medley, A., Kennedy, C., O'reilly, K. and Sweat, M. (2009) 'Effectiveness of peer education interventions for HIV prevention in developing countries: a systematic review and meta-analysis', *AIDS Education and Prevention*, vol 21, no 3, pp 181–206.

Michaelson, J. (2011) *Making it happen, wellbeing and the role of local government*, London: Local Government Association.

Milligan, C. and Fyfe, N.R. (2005) 'Preserving space for volunteers: exploring the links between voluntary welfare organisations, volunteering and citizenship', *Urban Studies*, vol 42, no 3, pp 417–33.

Minkler, M. (2004) 'Ethical challenges for the "outside" researcher in community-based participatory research', *Health Education & Behavior*, vol 31, no 6, pp 684–7.

Moewaka Barnes, H. (2000) 'Collaboration in community action: a successful partnership between indigenous communities and researchers', *Health Promotion International*, vol 15, no 1, pp 17–25.

Morgan, A. and Ziglio, E. (2007) 'Revitalising the evidence base for public health: an assets model', *Promotion & Education*, vol 14, supplement 2, pp 17–22.

Morgan, L.M. (2001) 'Community participation in health: perpetual allure, persistent challenge', *Health Policy and Planning*, vol 16, no 3, pp 221–30.

National Audit Office (2010) *Department of Health. Tackling inequalities in life expectancy in areas with the worst health and deprivation, Report by the Comptroller and Auditor General HC 186 Session 2010–2011*, London: National Audit Office.

National Institute for Health and Clinical Excellence (2006) 'Four commonly used methods to increase physical activity: brief interventions in primary care, exercise referral schemes, pedometers and community-based exercise programmes for walking and cycling', *Public Health Intervention Guidance*, London: National Institute for Health and Clinical Excellence.

National Institute for Health and Clinical Excellence (2008) 'Community engagement to improve health', *NICE public health guidance 9*, London: National Institute for Health and Clinical Excellence.

National Institute for Health and Clinical Excellence (2011) 'Increasing the uptake of HIV testing among men who have sex with men. Quick reference guide', *NICE Public Health Guidance*, London: National Institute for Health and Clinical Excellence.

Natural England (2011a) 'Key statistics'. Available at: http://www.wfh. naturalengland.org.uk/our-work/key-statistics

Natural England (2011b) 'Walking for Health'. Available at: http://www.wfh. naturalengland.org.uk/

Navarro, V. (ed) (2007) *Neoliberalism, globalization and inequalities: consequences for health and quality of life*, New York, NY: Baywood Publishing Company.

NCVO (National Council for Voluntary Organisations) Funding Commission (2010) *Funding the future: a 10-year framework for civil society*, London: National Council for Voluntary Organisations.

NEF (New Economics Foundation) Consulting (2010) *Catalysts for community action and investment: a Social Return on Investment analysis of community development work, based on a common outcomes framework. Executive summary*, London: Community Development Foundation.

Neighbourhood Renewal Unit (2003) *Factsheet 9. New Deal for Communities*, London: Office of the Deputy Prime Minister.

Neuberger, J. (1998) 'Primary care: core values, patients' priorities', *British Medical Journal*, vol 317, pp 260–2.

Neuberger, J. (2008) *Volunteering in the public services: health and social care. Baroness Neuberger's review as the Governments Volunteering Champion*, London: Cabinet Office, Office of the Third Sector.

NHS (National Health Service) Confederation and Altogether Better (2012) *Community Health Champions: creating new relationships with patients and communities*, London: NHS Confederation.

NHS Executive (1999) 'Patient and public involvement in the new NHS', HSC 1999/210.

NHS Future Forum (2011a) *Choice and competition. Delivering real choice. A report from the NHS Future Forum*, London: Department of Health.

NHS Future Forum (2011b) *Patient involvement and public accountability. A report from the NHS Future Forum*, London: Department of Health.

NHS Sheffield (no date) 'Introduction to Community Development and Health (ICDH)'. Available at: http://www.sheffield.nhs.uk/getinvolved/icdh.php

NICE Secretariat (2007) *Cost effectiveness vignettes for community engagement. A paper prepared by the NICE secretariat for the Community Engagement Programme.* Available from: www.nice.org.uk/nicemedia/live/11678/39722/39722.pdf

Nicholls, J., Lawlor, E.E.N. and Goodspeed, T. (2009) *A guide to Social Return on Investment*, London: Cabinet Office, NEF, Charities Evaluation Services, NVCO, New Philanthropy Capital.

Niyazi, F. and National Centre of Volunteering (1996) 'Involving volunteers from underrepresented groups', *Social policy research 105 – October 1996*, York: Joseph Rowntree Foundation.

Norris, S.L., Chowdhury, F.M., Van Le, K., Horsley, T., Brownstein, J.N., Zhang, X., Jack, L. and Satterfield, D.W. (2006) 'Effectiveness of community health workers in the care of persons with diabetes', *Diabetic Medicine*, vol 23, no 5, pp 544–56.

North, N. and Peckham, S. (2001) 'Analysing structural interests in primary care groups', *Social Policy and Administration*, vol 35, no 5, pp 426–40.

Nutbeam, D. (1998) 'Evaluating health promotion – progress, problems and solutions', *Health Promotion International*, vol 13, no 1, pp 27–44.

Oakley, A., Rajan, L. and Turner, H. (2002) 'Evaluating parent support initiatives: lessons from two case studies', *Health and Social Care in the Community*, vol 6, no 5, pp 318–30.

Oliver, M. (1997) 'The disability movement is a new social movement!', *Community Development Journal*, vol 32, no 3, pp 244–51.

Open Society Foundations (2011) *Roma health mediators: successes and challenges*, New York, NY: Open Society Foundations.

Opinion Leader Research (2001) 'A report on the findings from a listening exercise conducted with people from socially excluded groups evaluating the discussion documents: "Reforming the NHS complaints procedures", "Involving patients and the public in health care"', prepared for the Department of Health, Opinion Leader Research, London, October 2001.

Organisation for Economic Co-operation and Development (2011) 'Divided we stand: Why inequality keeps rising. Country note: United Kingdom'. Available at: www.oecd.org/social/socialpoliciesanddata/49170234.pdf

Parkin, S. and McKeganey, N. (2000) 'The rise and rise of peer education approaches', *Drugs: Education, Prevention and Policy*, vol 7, no 3, pp 293–310.

Peckham, S., Hunter, D. and Hann, A. (2008) 'The delivery and organization of public health in England: setting the research agenda', *Public Health*, vol 122, pp 99-104.

Perez-Escamilla, R., Hromi-Fiedler, A., Vega-Lopez, S., Bermudez-Millan, A. and Segura-Perez, S. (2008) 'Impact of peer nutrition education on dietary behaviors and health outcomes among Latinos: a systematic literature review', *Journal of Nutrition Education and Behavior*, vol 40, no 4, pp 208–25.

Petrack, E.M. (1984) 'Health care in Nicaragua: a social and historical perspective', *New York State Journal of Medicine*, vol 84, no 10, pp 523–5.

Petticrew, M. (2003) 'Why certain systematic reviews reach uncertain conclusions', *British Medical Journal*, vol 326, pp 756–8.

Phillips, A. and Rakusen, J. (1978) *Our bodies, ourselves: a health book by and for women*, London: Penguin Books.

Phillips, M. (2007) 'How welfarism is destroying Britain!', *Daily Mail*, 26 April.

PhORCAST (Public Health on line Resource for Careers Skills and Training) (no date) 'Non-medical public health specialists'. Available at: http://www.phorcast.org.uk/page.php?page_id=26

Plescia, M., Groblewski, M. and Chavis, L. (2006) 'A lay health advisor program to promote community capacity and change among change agents', *Health Promotion Practice*, vol 9, no 4, pp 434–9.

Pollock, A. and Price, D. (2011) 'How the secretary of state for health proposes to abolish the NHS in England', *British Medical Journal*, vol 342, no d1695.

Popay, J., Williams, G., Thomas, C. and Gatrell, A. (1998) 'Theorising inequalities in health: the place of lay knowledge', *Sociology of Health and Illness*, vol 20, no 5, pp 619–44.

Prentice, P. (2011) 'Welcome to the Big Society', *NMC Review*, vol 2, pp 4–7.

Public Administration Select Committee (2011) 'PASC launches inquiry into Government "Big Society" policy'. Available at: http://www.parliament.uk/business/committees/committees-a-z/commons-select/public-administration-select-committee/news/big-society-iq/

Public Health Resource Unit and Skills for Health (2008) *Public health skills and career framework*, Bristol: Skills for Health, Public Health Resource Unit, Skills for Business.

Rada, J., Ratima, M. and Howden-Chapman, P. (1999) 'Evidence-based purchasing of health promotion: methodology for reviewing evidence', *Health Promotion International*, vol 14, no 2, pp 177–87.

Rappaport, J. (1987) 'Terms of empowerment/exemplars of prevention: toward a theory for community psychology', *American Journal of Community Psychology*, vol 15, no 2, pp 121–48.

Realpe, A. and Wallace, L.M. (2010) *What is co-production?*, London: The Health Foundation.

Rhodes, S.D., Foley, K.L., Zometa, C.S. and Bloom, F.R. (2007) 'Lay health advisor interventions among Hispanics/Latinos: a qualitative systematic review', *American Journal of Preventive Medicine*, vol 33, no 5, pp 418–27.

Rifkin, S.B. (2001) 'Ten best readings on community participation and health', *African Health Sciences*, vol 1, no 1, pp 43–37.

Rifkin, S.B., Lewando-Hundt, G. and Draper, A.K. (2000) *Participatory approaches in health promotion and health planning. A literature review*, London: Health Development Agency.

Rogers, A., Bower, P., Gardner, C., Gateley, C., Kennedy, A., Lee, V., Middleton, P., Reeves, D. and Richardson, G. (2006) *The national evaluation of the pilot phase of the Expert Patients Programme. Final report*, Manchester: National Primary Care Research and Development Centre.

Rogers, B. and Robinson, E. (2004) *The benefits of community engagement. A review of evidence*, London: Active Citizenship Centre, Home Office.

Rognstad, M., Nortvedt, P. and Aasland, O. (2004) 'Helping motives in late modern society: values and attitudes among nursing students', *Nursing Ethics*, vol 11, no 3, pp 227–39.

Rosenthal, E.L., Wiggins, N., Brownstein, J.N., Johnson, S., Borbon, I.A. and Rael, R. (1998) *The final report of the National Community Health Advisor Study*, Tucson, AZ: The University of Arizona.

Ross, M.W., Harzke, A.J., Scott, D.P., Mccann, K. and Kelley, M. (2006) 'Outcomes of project wall talk: an HIV/AIDS peer education program implemented within the Texas state prison system', *AIDS Education and Prevention*, vol 18, no 6, pp 504–17.

Rudolf, M.C.J., Christie, D., Mcelhone, S., Sahota, P., Dixey, R., Walker, J. and Wellings, C. (2006) Watch it: a community based programme for obese children and adolescents', *Archives of Disease in Childhood*, vol 91, pp 736–9.

Ryan-Collins, J., Sanfilippo, L. and Spratt, S. (2007) *Unintended consequences. How the efficiency agenda erodes local public services and a new public benefit model to restore them*, London: New Economics Foundation.

Rychetnik, L., Frommer, M., Hawe, P. and Shiell, A. (2002) 'Criteria for evaluating evidence on public health interventions', *Journal of Epidemiology and Community Health*, vol 56, no 2, pp 119–27.

Sang, B. (2004) 'Choice, participation and accountability: assessing the potential impact of legislation promoting patient and public involvement in health in the UK', *Health Expectations*, vol 7, no 3, pp 187–190.

Schofield, S. (no date) 'Local sufficiency'. Available at: http://www.lessnet.co.uk/sufficiency1.html

Scott-Samuel, A. and Springett, J. (2007) 'Hegemony or health promotion? Prospects for reviving England's lost discipline', *The Journal of the Royal Society for the Promotion of Health*, vol 127, no 5, pp 211–14.

Secretary of State for Communities and Local Government (2008) *Communities in control: real people, real power*, Cm 7427, London: Department for Communities and Local Government.

Secretary of State for Health (1999) *Saving lives: our healthier nation*, Cm 4386, London: The Stationery Office.

Secretary of State for Health (2006) *Our health, our care, our say: a new direction for community services*, Cm 6732, London: The Stationery Office.

Secretary of State for Health (2010a) *Equity and excellence: liberating the NHS*, Cm 7881, London: The Stationery Office.

Secretary of State for Health (2010b) *Healthy lives, healthy people: our strategy for public health in England*, CM7985, London: HM Government.

Sheffield Well-Being Consortium (no date[a]) 'Community Health Champions'. Available at: http://sheffieldwellbeing.org.uk/contracts-projects/community-health-champions

Sheffield Well-Being Consortium (no date[b]) *Community Health Champions: tell their stories*, Sheffield: Sheffield Well-being Consortium.

Shields, L. and Watson, R. (2007) 'The demise of nursing in the UK: a warning for medicine', *Journal of the Royal Society of Medicine*, vol 100, no 2, pp 70–4.

Shiner, M. (1999) 'Defining peer education', *Journal of Adolescence*, vol 22, no 4, pp 555–66.

Shircore, R. (2009) *Guide for world class commissioners. Promoting health and well-being: reducing inequalities*, London: Royal Society for Public Health.

Smith, R.D. and Petticrew, M. (2010) 'Public health evaluation in the twenty-first century: time to see the wood as well as the trees', *Journal of Public Health*, vol 32, no 1, pp 2–7.

Smithies, J. and Webster, G. (eds) (1998) *Community involvement in health: from passive recipients to active participants*, Aldershot: Ashgate Publishing.

Social Exclusion Unit (2001) *A new commitment to neighbourhood renewal. National strategy action plan*, London: Cabinet Office.

Social Market Foundation (no date) 'About the Social Market Foundation'. Available at: http://www.smf.co.uk/about

South, J. and Sahota, P. (2010) 'Harnessing people power in health promotion', *Primary Health Care*, vol 20, no 8, pp 16–21.

South, J., Woodward, J. and Lowcock, D. (2007) 'New beginnings: stakeholder perspectives on the role of health trainers', *The Journal of the Royal Society for the Promotion of Health*, vol 127, no 5, pp 224–30.

South, J., Meah, A. and Branney, P. (2009) *People in public health. Expert hearings: a summary report*, Leeds: Centre for Health Promotion Research, Leeds Metropolitan University.

South, J., Branney, P., White, J. and Gamsu, M. (2010a) *Engaging the public in delivering health improvement: research briefing*, Leeds: Centre for Health Promotion Research, Leeds Metropolitan University.

South, J., Meah, A., Bagnall, A.-M., Kinsella, K., Branney, P., White, J. and Gamsu, M. (2010b) 'People in public health – a study of approaches to develop and support people in public health roles', report for the National Institute for Health Research Service Delivery and Organisation Programme. Available at: www.netscc.ac.uk/hsdr/files/project/SDO_FR_08-1716-206_V01.pdf

South, J., Raine, G. and White, J. (2010c) *Community Health Champions: evidence review*, Leeds: Centre for Health Promotion Research, Leeds Metropolitan University.

South, J., Branney, P. and Kinsella, K. (2011a) 'Citizens bridging the gap? Interpretations of volunteering roles in two public health projects', *Voluntary Sector Review*, vol 2, no 3, pp 297–315.

South, J., Kinsella, K., Giuntoli, G., Mckenna, J., Long, J. and Carless, D. (2011b) 'Walking for health: a qualitative study of links between community engagement, social capital and health outcomes within volunteer-led health walks', 'Bridging the gap between science and practice', 3rd conference and 7th annual meeting of HEPA Europe, Amsterdam.

South, J., Meah, A. and Branney, P. (2011c) '"Think differently and be prepared to demonstrate trust": findings from public hearings, England, on supporting lay people in public health roles', *Health Promotion International*, vol 27, no 2, pp 284–94.

South, J., Kinsella, K. and Meah, A. (2012) 'Lay perspectives on lay health worker roles, boundaries and participation within three UK community-based health promotion projects', *Health Education Research*, vol 27, no 4, pp 656–70.

South, J., Meah, A., Bagnall, A.-M. and Jones, R. (forthcoming) 'Dimensions of lay health worker programmes: results of a scoping study and production of a descriptive framework', *Global Health Promotion*.

Springett, J. (2001) 'Participatory approaches to evaluation in health promotion', in Goodstadt, M.S., Hyndman, B., Mcqueen, D., Potvin, L., Rootman, I. and Springett, J. (eds) *Evaluation in health promotion. Principles and perspectives*, Denmark: WHO Europe, pp 83–105.

Springett, J., Owens, C. and Callaghan, J. (2007) 'The challenge of combining "lay" knowledge with "evidenced-based" practice in health promotion: Fag Ends Smoking Cessation Service', *Critical Public Health*, vol 17, no 3, pp 243–56.

Stevens, P.E. (1994) 'HIV prevention education for lesbians and bisexual women: a cultural analysis of a community intervention', *Social Science and Medicine*, vol 39, no 11, pp 1565–78.

Stuckler, D., Basu, S., Suhrcke, M., Coutts, A. and Mckee, M. (2011) 'Effects of the 2008 recession on health: a first look at European data', *The Lancet*, vol 378, pp 124–5.

Sullivan, H., Barnes, M. and Matka, E. (2006) 'Collaborative capacity and strategies in area-based initiatives', *Public Administration*, vol 84, no 2, pp 289–310.

Swider, S.M. (2002) 'Outcome effectiveness of community health workers: an integrative literature review', *Public Health Nursing*, vol 19, no 1, pp 11–20.

Taylor, B., Mathers, J., Atfield, T. and Parry, J. (2011) 'Thesis: what are the challenges to the Big Society in maintaining lay involvement in health improvement, and how can they be met?', *Journal of Public Health*, vol 33, no 1, pp 5–10.

Taylor, P. (2003) 'The lay contribution to public health', in Orme, J., Powell, J., Taylor, P., Harrison, T. and Grey, M. (eds) *Public health for the 21st century. New perspectives on policy, participation and practice*, Berkshire: Open University Press, pp 128–44.

Taylor, T., Serrano, E. and Anderson, J. (2001) 'Management issues related to effectively implementing a nutrition education program using peer educators', *Journal of Nutrition Education*, vol 33, no 5, pp 284–92.

Taylor-Goodby, P. (ed) (2009) *Reframing social citizenship*, Oxford: Oxford University Press.

Teasdale, S. (2008) *In good health: assessing the impact of volunteering in the NHS*, London: Institute for Volunteering Research, NAVSM.

The Asset-Based Community Development Institute (no date) 'Homepage'. Available at: http://www.abcdinstitute.org/

The Commission on the Future of Volunteering (2008) *Report of the Commission on the Future of Volunteering and Manifesto for Change*, London: The Commission on the Future of Volunteering, Volunteering England.

The Countryside Agency (2005) *Walking the way to health 2000–2005 summary of local health walk evaluations*, Cheltenham: The Countryside Agency.

The King's Fund (2011) *The future of leadership and management in the NHS: no more heroes*, London: The King's Fund.

The Marmot Review (2010a) *Fair society, healthy lives. The Marmot Review, strategic review of health inequalities in England post-2010*, London: The Marmot Review.

The Marmot Review (2010b) *Fair society, healthy lives. The Marmot Review. Executive summary, strategic review of health inequalities in England post-2010*, London: The Marmot Review.

The Telegraph (2011) 'Inflation rise to land Coalition with bumper benefits bill', 18 October.

Tones, K. and Tilford, S. (eds) (2001) *Health promotion: effectiveness, efficiency and equity*, Cheltenham: Nelson Thornes.

Trayers, T. and Lawlor, D.A. (2007) 'Bridging the gap in health inequalities with the help of health trainers: a realistic task in hostile environments? A short report for debate', *Journal of Public Health*, vol 29, no 3, pp 218–221.

TUC (Trades Union Congress) (2009) 'New charter aims to strengthen ties between volunteers and staff'. Available at: http://www.tuc.org.uk/union/tuc-17328-f0.cfm

Turner, D. and Powell, T. (2011) *NHS commissioning standard note: SN/SP/5607*, London: Library, House of Commons.

Turning Point (2010) *Citizen advisors. Linking services and empowering communities*, London: Turning Point.

US Department of Health and Human Services, Health Resources and Services Administration and Bureau of Health Professions (2007) *Community health worker national workforce study*, Washington, DC: US Department of Health and Human Services.

Veenstra, G. (2000) 'Social capital, SES and health: an individual-level analysis', *Social Science & Medicine*, vol 50, no 5, pp 619–29.

Vidal, J. (2011) 'Why are the big emitters gambling with all our fates?', *The Guardian*, 25 November.

Visram, S. and Drinkwater, C. (2005) *Health trainers. A review of the evidence*, Newcastle: The Primary Care Development Centre, University of Northumbria.

Volunteering England (no date) *Seeing is believing. Volunteer involvement in health and social care*, London: Volunteering England.

Volunteering England (2011) 'Volunteering and state benefit – some more myths busted'. Available at: www.volunteering.org.uk/WhatWeDo/Policy/Policy+blog/Volunteering+and+state+benefits+-+some+more+myths+busted

Volunteering England (2012) 'What is volunteering?'. Available at: http://www.volunteering.org.uk/iwanttovolunteer/what-is-volunteering

Volunteering England and TUC (2009) 'A charter for strengthening relations between paid staff and volunteers'. Available at: http://www.tuc.org.uk/workplace/tuc-17329-f0.cfm

Walking for Health Team Natural England (2011) *Guidance note 5. Training and support*, Cheltenham: Natural England.

Wallerstein, N. (1992) 'Powerlessness, empowerment, and health: implications for health promotion programs', *American Journal of Health Promotion*, vol 6, no 3, pp 197–205.

Wallerstein, N. (2002) 'Empowerment to reduce health disparities', *Scandinavian Journal of Public Health*, vol 30, no 59, pp 72–7.

Wallerstein, N. (2006) *What is the evidence on effectiveness of empowerment to improve health?*, Copenhagen: WHO Regional Office for Europe (Health Evidence Network report).

Walt, G. (ed) (1990) *Community health workers in national programmes: just another pair of hands?*, Milton Keynes: Open University Press.

Wanless, D. (2002) *Securing our future health: taking a long-term view*, London: HM Treasury.

Wanless, D. (2004) *Securing good health for the whole population. Final report*, London: HM Treasury.

Ware, P. and Todd, M.J. (2002) 'British statutory sector partnerships with the voluntary sector: exploring rhetoric and reality', *The Social Policy Journal*, vol 1, no 3, pp 5–20.

Watkins, E.L., Harlan, C., Eng, E. and Gansky, S.A. (1994) 'Assessing the effectiveness of lay health advisors with migrant farmworkers', *Family & Community Health*, vol 16, no 4, pp 72–87.

Watt, G. (2002) 'The inverse care law today', *The Lancet*, vol 360, no 9328, pp 252–4.

Watt, R.G., Mcglone, P., Russell, J.J., Tull, K.I. and Dowler, E. (2006) 'The process of establishing, implementing and maintaining a social support infant feeding programme', *Public Health Nutrition*, vol 9, no 6, pp 714–21.

Wei, N.M. (2010) *Hansard*, col 1012, 16 June, House of Lords.

Westhoff, M.H. and Hopman-Rock, M. (2002) 'Dissemination and implementation of "Aging Well and Healthily": a health-education and exercise program for older adults', *Journal of Aging & Physical Activity*, vol 10, no 4, pp 382–95.

White, J. and Kinsella, K. (2011) *Scarborough Health Trainer Service: evaluation report for the period January to October 2010*, Leeds: Centre for Health Promotion Research, Leeds Metropolitan University.

White, J. and South, J. (2012) 'Health trainers can help people manage long-term conditions', *Primary Health Care*, vol 22, no 2, pp 26–31.

White, J., South, J. and Kinsella, K. (2010a) *The North Lincolnshire Health Trainer Service 2009–10: an evaluation*, Leeds: Centre for Health Promotion Research, Leeds Metropolitan University.

White, J., South, J., Woodall, J. and Kinsella, K. (2010b) *Altogether Better thematic evaluation – Community Health Champions and empowerment*, Leeds: Centre for Health Promotion, Leeds Metropolitan University.

White, J., Kinsella, K. and South, J. (2011) *An evaluation of social prescribing health trainers in South and West Bradford*, Leeds: Centre for Health Promotion Research, Leeds Metropolitan University.

Whitehead, M. (2007) 'A typology of actions to tackle social inequalities in health', *Journal of Epidemiology and Community Health*, vol 61, no 6, pp 473–8.

Whitehead, M. (2010) 'The right wood, but barking up the wrong tree', *Journal of Public Health*, vol 32, no 1, pp 16–17.

Wilkinson, R. and Marmot, M. (eds) (2003) *Social determinants of health: the solid facts* (2nd edn), Denmark: World Health Organization Europe.

Wilkinson, R. and Pickett, K. (eds) (2009) *The spirit level: why equality is better for everyone*, London: Penguin Books.

Williamson, L.M., Hart, G.J., Flowers, P., Frankis, J.S. and Der, G.J. (2001) 'The Gay Men's Task Force: the impact of peer education on the sexual health behaviour of homosexual men in Glasgow', *Sexually Transmitted Infections*, vol 77, no 6, pp 427–32.

Wilson, F. and Mabhala, M. (eds) (2009) *Key concepts in public health*, London: SAGE.

Wilson, J. (2000) 'Volunteering', *Annual Review of Sociology*, vol 26, pp 215–40.

Wilson, R., Leach, M., Henman, O., Tam, H. and Ukkonen, J. (2011) *Civic limits: how much more involved can people get?*, London: ResPublica.

Witmer, A., Seifer, S.D., Finocchio, L., Leslie, J. and O Neil, E.H. (1995) 'Community health workers: integral members of the health care work force', *Amercian Journal of Public Health*, vol 85, no 8 (part 1), pp 1055–8.

World Health Organization (1978) 'Declaration of Alma-Ata. International Conference on Primary Health Care, Alma-Ata, USSR, 6–12 September'. Available at: http://www.euro.who.int/en/who-we-are/policy-documents/declaration-of-alma-ata,-1978

World Health Organization (1981) *Global strategy for health for all by the year 2000*, Geneva: World Health Organization.

World Health Organization (1986) *Ottawa Charter for health promotion*, Geneva: World Health Organization.

World Health Organization (1987) 'Community health workers: pillars of health for all', Report of the Interregional Conference 1986, Yaoundé, Cameroon: World Health Organization, unpublished document SHS/CIH/87.2.

World Health Organization (2002) 'Community participation in local health and sustainable development. Approaches and techniques', *European sustainable development and health series no. 4*, Copenhagen: WHO Regional Office for Europe.

World Health Organization (2007) *Community health workers: what do we know about them*, Geneva: World Health Organization.

World Health Organization (2008a) *Closing the gap in a generation. Health equity through action on the social determinants of health. Final report, executive summary*, Geneva: Commission on Social Determinants of Health.

World Health Organization (2008b) *The World Health Report 2008. Primary health care – now more than ever*, Geneva: World Health Organization.

World Health Organization (2009) *Milestones in health promotion: statements from global conferences*, Geneva: World Health Organization.

World Health Organization (2011) 'Rio political declaration on social determinants of health', World Conference on Social Determinants of Health, Rio de Janeiro, Brazil.

World Health Organization Regional Office for Europe (2011) 'Governance for health in the 21st century: a study conducted for the WHO Regional Office for Europe'. Available at: http://www.euro.who.int/__data/assets/pdf_file/0010/148951/RC61_InfDoc6.pdf

World Health Organization Regional Office for Europe (2012) 'The new European policy for health – Health 2020: vision, values, main directions and approaches'. Available at: http://www.euro.who.int/__data/assets/pdf_file/0007/147724/wd09E_Health2020_111332.pdf

Year of Care (2011) *Thanks for the petunias – a guide to developing and commissioning non-traditional providers to support the self management of people with long term conditions*, NHS Diabetes.

Yorkshire and Humber Regional Health Trainer Hub (2011) *Evidence briefing no 1, behaviour change for health: the health trainer approach*, Leeds: Leeds Metropolitan University.

Zhang, D. and Unschuld, P.U. (2008) 'China's barefoot doctor: past, present, and future', *The Lancet*, vol 372, no 9653, pp 1865–7.

Ziersch, A., Gaffney, J. and Tomlinson, D.R. (2000) 'STI prevention and the male sex industry in London: evaluating a pilot peer education programme', *Sexually Transmitted Infections*, vol 76, no 6, pp 447–53.

Appendix:
The People in Public Health study

The People in Public Health study sought to bring greater clarity around the different models in practice and to determine how public health services could support lay people involved in delivering public health programmes. The aims of the study were:

- to improve understanding of valid approaches to identifying, developing and supporting lay people who take on public health roles in community-based public health activities;
- to undertake research on public perspectives regarding the acceptability and value of lay people in public health roles; and
- to aid public health commissioning and planning by identifying elements of good practice and how these might be applied to different contexts.

A research partnership between Leeds Metropolitan University, NHS Bradford and Airedale (a teaching Primary Care Trust), and the Regional Public Health Group, Government Office for Yorkshire and Humber was responsible for the implementation of the study, although the study was national in scope. This collaborative approach enabled the research team to maximise dialogue with the public health field in England and to promote shared learning. The study was conducted in two distinct phases over a 27-month period (2007–09). The first phase comprised a scoping study with three linked elements:

- A systematic scoping review of 224 publications on lay engagement in public health roles that mapped models occurring in public health practice and thematic issues for service delivery and organisation.
- Three expert hearings where key informants with relevant experience and expertise presented evidence. Deliberative methods were used to explore different perspectives and stimulate debate on contested issues.
- The establishment of a Register of Interest where information about projects involving lay health workers could be posted combined with some follow-up site visits to current projects.

Phase 2 involved primary qualitative research to investigate roles and support issues in greater depth through five case studies of public health projects. The case studies each reflected a different model of practice and community of interest (see Table A1). Interviews were conducted with a range of stakeholders involved in the case study projects, including public health commissioners, practitioners, partner organisations, lay health workers, volunteers and programme recipients. In total, 136 people took part in interviews and focus groups. The results were

Table A1: Case study sites

Case study	Model	Target group	Public health focus	Lead delivery organisation
Sexual health outreach	Peer education	Men who have sex with men	Sexual health (uptake of screening)	Voluntary sector
Walking for Health (local scheme)	Peer support (independent)	All population groups	Physical activity	NHS
Breastfeeding peer support	Peer support (service-linked)	Parents	Nutrition (breastfeeding)	Third sector
Community Health Educators	Bridging	All population groups	Nutrition Physical activity	Voluntary sector
Neighbourhood health project	Community organising	All population groups	Health and well-being	Local authority

Source: South et al (2010, p 147).

analysed and a series of case study reports were generated. This was followed by a cross–case analysis to identify patterns across the five cases. At the end of the study, findings from Phase 1 and 2 were brought together and recommendations were made for policy, practice and research (for more detail, see final report [South et al, 2010b]).

The People in Public Health study was funded by the National Institute for Health Research Service Delivery and Organisation Programme (project number 08/1716/206). The Service Delivery and Organisation Programme has since merged with the Health Services Research programme to form the National Institute for Health Research Health Services and Delivery Research, where the full report can be accessed. The views and opinions expressed in this book are those of the authors and do not necessarily reflect those of the NHS, NIHR or the Department of Health.

Index

Note: The following abbreviations have been used – f = figure; n = note; t = table